**The Handbook
of Midwifery
Research**

The Handbook of Midwifery Research

Mary Steen

Professor of Midwifery, Faculty of Health & Social Care, University of Chester

Taniya Roberts

Senior Lecturer, Midwifery, Faculty of Health & Social Care, University of Chester

WILEY-BLACKWELL

A John Wiley & Sons, Ltd., Publication

Library of Congress Cataloging-in-Publication Data
Steen, Mary.
 The handbook of midwifery research / Mary Steen, Taniya Roberts
  p. ; cm.
 Includes bibliographical references and index.
 ISBN 978-1-4051-9510-2 (pbk. : alk. paper)
 1. Midwifery–Research–Handbooks, manuals, etc. I. Roberts, Taniya. II. Title.
 [DNLM: 1. Midwifery–methods–Handbooks. 2. Research Design–Handbooks. WQ 165]
 RG950.S74 2011
 618.20072–dc22

                                                        2010041326

A catalogue record for this book is available from the British Library.

1   2011

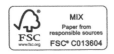

Contents

Foreword

As the UK government is beginning to recognise, encouraging an increasing synergy between practice and research is essential to maximise the quality of care, and the development and retention of staff. The recent institution of the NIHR Fellowship awards in the UK is an indication of this intent. However, I am very conscious from my teaching of research methods to undergraduate midwives that it is, generally, the last module they want to do. Most people who want to become midwives are deeply drawn to practice. Many have waited for years to be able to get on to a midwifery course, and they are highly focused on getting through their course, and into practice. Research seems to be a distant irrelevance. Despite this, many of these same students after some years in practice find that they have an increasing number of questions that they would really like to have an answer for. Some of these emerge through clinical experience, and some are borne of frustration at the way things are being done, or at policies and procedures that do not seem to make sense to them, or for the women babies and families they are attending. There are also some students who are curious about aspects of midwifery even during their training.

For student midwives, and for qualified staff who are beginning to turn towards this possibility, there is a plethora of books relating advanced aspects of research, often with a focus on specific qualitative or quantitative techniques. For many of those braving the research ocean for the first time, these books can be very dense and off-putting. Terms like theoretical perspective, epistemology, ontology, and etic and emic perspectives are profoundly scary. This book, in contrast, provides a clear and straightforward introduction to the whole spectrum of research in maternity care. The authors have broken the process down into easy steps, and provided a clear overview at each stage, with reassuringly familiar examples of how the knowledge they present might be applied in practice. For those just dipping their toes in the cool waters of research this text provides easy access to the warm shallows. Even for those who are more familiar, there are insights to be gained from reading through the book. I hope you enjoy reading it as much as I did!

Soo Downe
Director, ReaCH (Research in Childbirth and Health) Unit
University of Central Lancashire

Preface

Research is a subject in its own right and initially many midwives and students will be overwhelmed by the whole process of how to understand and undertake research. The initial idea of writing this book arose when the authors gained an insight into how some midwives were finding it difficult, first, to understand how to search and make sense of research evidence and, second, how to write a research proposal and, finally, how to undertake a research study. In addition, some student midwives reported similar concerns and this did nothing for their confidence to undertake research.

This instigated the authors to write a handbook on understanding and undertaking research which aims to reduce the difficulties some midwives and students have discussed and to promote confidence to undertake research. The authors, therefore, feel there is a need for a handbook which specifically focuses on the needs of midwives and students, which gives midwifery-led research examples, is written in a clear and concise way to help increase their knowledge and clarify some of the misunderstandings reported.

The book is organised into two parts:

Part I Understanding research
Part II Undertaking research

This book will, hopefully help support midwives and students to gain knowledge, skills and increase their confidence to undertake research successfully and to not stop there! The final chapter will focus on encouraging midwives and students to write an article for publication or give a conference presentation on their research work. The authors will draw upon their own and other midwives' personal experiences of understanding and undertaking midwifery research. The authors will also refer to some midwifery studies successfully completed as examples. Both qualitative and quantitative examples will be included and this will help midwives gain confidence to undertake research themselves. Remember, the authors had to start somewhere and have acquired research knowledge and skills over a number of years and now they want to inspire midwives and students to do the same.

Research terminology in itself can be confusing and knowledge of new words and their meanings will need to be learnt whilst trying to understand

and undertake research. A useful glossary of research words and terms is included in this handbook.

Research informs and links midwifery education, policy, management and practice. It is, therefore, vitally important that midwives are able to understand what research is, how to find the evidence and how to critique both qualitative and quantitative evidence, so they can make sense of the evidence upon which to base their care and practice. Midwives will then be able to undertake research, either as a team member of a collaborative research study or as a principal or chief investigator of midwifery-led research studies.

It is also vitally important that student midwives develop the knowledge and skills to understand research and for some to become researchers who will have the ability, confidence and passion to undertake midwifery research. Student midwives are our future; it is vital that they develop the competences and confidence to understand and undertake research as this will empower and enable them to promote evidence-based practice, further develop midwifery as a profession and increase the likelihood of women, their babies and their families receiving the best care possible which will be based on research evidence.

About the book

Part I starts with a chapter on *Introduction to midwifery research* which sets the scene and covers an understanding of the general principles of research, the importance of the research question, the approaches that can be undertaken, the differences between these and the importance of applying evidence to midwifery practice. Chapter 2, *Finding the evidence*, explains in detail how to undertake a literature review, the sources of evidence available and how to use a search strategy, and gives useful examples. In addition, midwifery-related structured and systematic reviews are described and discussed in an attempt to promote a better understanding of how to undertake these aspects of research. Chapter 3, *Making sense of the evidence*, covers the critiquing aspects of research evidence, gives an insight into how evidence is graded and clearly differentiates the differences between qualitative and quantitative approaches.

Part II focuses on how to undertake research and includes four chapters. *Data collection techniques* cover both qualitative and quantitative methods and are the focus of Chapter 4. This chapter gives specific details on how to undertake a research interview and how to design a questionnaire as these will be the most likely data collection techniques a midwife or student will make use of. Chapter 5, *Ethics and research governance*, introduces the role of ethics when undertaking research and discusses the importance of research governance. Ethical issues relating to midwifery research are considered and specific details on how to obtain ethical approval are addressed to help midwives and students achieve this successfully. *Data analysis* is the focus of Chapter 6. An introduction to data analysis, which is followed by specific sections of both qualitative and quantitative analysis methods, is covered and a basic understanding of statistics is also included to help midwives and students link the type of data collected with the appropriate statistical test required to analyse a specific type of data (fit for purpose). Finally, *the research dissertation/thesis and dissemination* are the focus of Chapter 7. Writing skills and how to structure your dissertation/thesis are described and discussed. Guidelines and advice on how to get your work published and presenting a conference paper are given. A specific section on useful resources and becoming a researcher brings the book to a close.

About the authors

Professor Mary Steen RGN, RM, BHSc, PGCRM, PG Dip HE, MCGI, PhD

Mary was appointed as a Professor of Midwifery at the University of Chester in 2010. She has been a practising midwife for over 23 years and been involved in midwifery research since 1990. During that time she has become very interested in a wide remit of midwifery and family health issues which has led her to undertake several research studies and service development projects; with the overall aim to improve the care and services for women, babies and their families. Her PhD research focused specifically on the care and consequences of perineal trauma after childbirth and following laboratory experiments, focus group interviews and undertaking two randomised controlled trials she invented a new localised cooling treatment (femepad) to alleviate perineal pain. She has published her work in several health-related journals, presented at national and international conferences and written book chapters and books. She has contributed to books entitled *Ask a Midwife*, *Pregnancy Day by Day* and is the author of a recently published book *Pregnancy and Birth: Everything you Need to Know.*

She is the programme leader for an undergraduate research dissertation module, supervises Masters and PhD students and an external examiner for the MSc in Midwifery at Trinity College, Dublin. She is the professional editor of the Royal College of Midwives magazine and student e-zine, a peer reviewer for several journals and funding bodies. Her work has received several awards for clinical innovation, original research and outstanding services to midwifery. Mary continues to be involved in midwifery practice and particularly enjoys teaching antenatal and postnatal exercises, active birth, attending home births and then supporting parents through the transition to parenthood

Taniya Roberts RGN, RM, BSc (Hons), MSc, PG Dip PE

Taniya has been qualified as a midwife for over 18 years and her midwifery practice has included being a hospital and a team midwife at the Homerton Hospital, London and a hospital midwife at St Michael's Hospital, Bristol. Prior to becoming a midwife, Taniya had been a Night Sister at the Royal

London Hospital in the late 1980s and this led her to develop a keen interest in women's health; she took a subsequent course in gynaecological nursing, and this resulted in a post as a Research Sister. She ultimately progressed into midwifery practice and qualified as a midwife in 1992.

She has been involved in research since the early 1990s when she was Research Sister in Ovarian Cancer Screening at King's College Hospital, London. In 1995 she took up a position as Specialist Midwife Practitioner in Fetal Echocardiography at Guy's Hospital, London, which was the only position of its kind within the UK. In 2002 she became a Midwifery researcher at St. Michael's Hospital, Bristol, where she led a qualitative study on women's experiences of obstetric emergencies and participated in a quantitative study on fetal and maternal heart rate monitoring. She has published on a number of research-related topics and most recently has published a series of articles on understanding phenomenology, grounded theory and ethnography. Taniya is also a peer reviewer for an international journal on research methodologies.

Since 2004, Taniya has been a Senior Lecturer in the Department of Midwifery and Reproductive Health, Faculty of Health and Social Care, University of Chester. She has a particular passion for teaching research and is the module leader for the Context of Research module for third-year midwifery students.

Taniya is also module leader for several other midwifery-specific modules. She is a Link Lecturer to a maternity unit and a gynaecological nursing ward. She is currently studying for a PhD and undertaking a Heideggerian Hermeneutic Phenomenological study of midwives' experiences of caring for women with a raised BMI of 30> during the childbirth process.

Acknowledgements

Andrea McLaughlin (Head of Midwifery and Reproductive Health) at the University of Chester for her support and proof reading of the chapters. Louise Simpson (Practice Development Midwife), Clare Mather (Delivery Suite Co-ordinator/Advanced Practitioner) at Mid-Cheshire Hospitals NHS Foundation Trust and Gillian Hughes (Senior Lecturer in Midwifery) at the University of Chester for kindly giving their permission to use as examples a covering letter and data collection tools (interview guides and a survey questionnaire) from their Master's theses.

Duncan Greaves and Paul Roberts, the authors' supportive, patient and understanding husbands. A special thanks to Theresa Holgate (data analyst) and Dr Paul Marchant (statistician), whose advice was sought to assist with some statistical examples.

Acknowledgements

Part I

Understanding research

1 Introduction to midwifery research

Introducing research

The focus of this chapter is to introduce midwifery research, types of knowledge, audit and research, the differences between qualitative and quantitative research and the importance of evidence-based practice. This chapter will assist midwives and students to gain basic knowledge and understanding of what research is and why it is important. This new knowledge will enable midwives and students to understand and appreciate the need for evidence-based practice when caring for childbearing women, their babies and their families. The importance of evidence-based practice will be stressed to promote good standards of care.

Aim

To introduce midwives and students to different research approaches that will help them develop an understanding of types of knowledge, the differences between audit and research and the importance of evidence-based practice.

Learning outcomes

By the end of this introductory chapter, midwives and students:

- will be able to recognise different types of knowledge;
- will be able to distinguish between qualitative and quantitative approaches;
- will know the difference between audit and research;
- will understand the importance of evidence-based practice.

Research questions – what, where, when, why, who and how?

When undertaking research, you firstly have to ask yourself the questions what, where, when, why, who and how? This will help you decide the research approach you need to apply, either quantitative (measures/numbers/counts/frequencies) or qualitative (understanding of words/phrases/language). It

The Handbook of Midwifery Research, First Edition. Mary Steen and Taniya Roberts.
© 2011 Mary Steen and Taniya Roberts. Published 2011 by Blackwell Publishing Ltd.

will also help you to develop a research question or hypothesis (theory) that needs asking and is relevant to something you are curious or concerned about in midwifery education, policy, management or practice. The first task, when you have an idea of the research question you would like to ask, is to find out about any existing evidence there is available on the subject matter.

Ideally, you should choose something you are passionate about or some burning issue you would like to address. Once you have made a decision about what you would like to investigate or explore and have a preliminary research question, you will need to undertake a literature search to see if the research question has already been asked or not. Using a search strategy and structuring the review in some way (which is covered in the next chapter) can be helpful in organising the evidence or identifying a lack of evidence you may find. The search strategy and literature review can be influenced by the research approach adopted and this chapter introduces the different approaches to research.

Midwifery and research

Midwifery-led research has not had a long history, in fact as late as the 1980s there was a paucity of research in this area. Some early midwifery research studies, such as the routine shaving of women in labour (Romney, 1980), the routine use of enemas during labour (Romney & Gordon, 1981), the use of episiotomies (Sleep *et al.*, 1984) and the routine admission of women in labour (Garforth & Garcia, 1987), are examples of traditional midwifery practices that were found to be of little benefit to women. The publication of *Effective Care in Pregnancy and Childbirth*, which provided details of several systematic reviews, initially assisted in the dissemination of research evidence to the midwifery profession (Chalmers *et al.*, 1989).

The Midwifery Research Database (MIRIAD) had 393 studies recorded in 1995, whereas at its inception period, 1976–1980, only 21 studies were recorded (McCormick & Renfrew, 1997). Presently it is difficult to determine exactly how many midwifery studies are in the public domain, but an internet search using the term 'UK midwifery research studies' on Google Scholar resulted in 38 800 hits (not all necessarily research studies); this does suggest that the body of knowledge has increased significantly. More midwives are now in possession of PhDs, both in the academic and clinical environments, and this means that they have conducted a significant and valid research study.

It was not until the 1980s that the concept of research was included in the midwifery curriculum (Macdonald, 2004). Since then it has become an integral element to student midwives' studies with assignments being based on research critiques or the formulation of research proposals. Post-registration students who are studying at Master's level in most universities have to conduct and write up their research study as part of their dissertation.

Students can add to the body of knowledge of midwifery by conducting a research study. An understanding of the research process is therefore essential from an academic viewpoint. However, it is not the academic viewpoint, but

Box 1.1 The Code: Standards of conduct, performance and ethics for nurses and midwives (NMC, 2008, p. 4).

- Provide a high standard of practice and care at all times.
- Use the best available evidence.
- You must deliver care based on the best available evidence or best practice.
- You must ensure any advice you give is evidence based if you are suggesting healthcare products or service.

---

evidence-based clinical practice that drives this educational research awareness. In the UK the Nursing and Midwifery Council (NMC) Code (2008), states that practice and care should be underpinned by the best available evidence (Box 1.1).

Types of research knowledge

As mentioned previously a process needs to be followed and this starts with trying to determine 'what you want to know'. This sounds easy, but the reality is that this starting point does take time. It is your thinking time, time to put your thoughts into reality. What burning issues do you want to address? What subject or topic are you passionate about? What have you observed in practice that merits further research? At the beginning of each research module, these are the questions we put to the students and the response we usually receive from them is 'it's not as easy as you think'. Rees (2003) refers to this as the 'conceptual phase', where the potential researcher, or in this case the student, embarking on a research proposal is trying to determine 'what they want to know' and to refine that further into 'how do I find out what I want to know'; and so the research process begins.

The next step is trying to work out how you are going to go about obtaining that information. You might want to find out about people's feelings, experiences of events or circumstances, such as *Women's experiences of obstetric emergencies* (Mapp & Hudson, 2005); or how an intervention/treatment can improve care, e.g. *Ice packs and cooling gel pads* versus *no localised treatment for relief of perineal pain: a randomised controlled trial* (Steen & Marchant, 2007). Or you might have a general idea but want the focus/theory of the study to be generated by the information you collect (Furber & Thomson, 2006).

The type of knowledge that you want to obtain then determines the type of research approach that you will follow which is also referred to as a research paradigm (or the 'philosophical underpinnings'!). This essentially refers to the school of thought or beliefs which forms the basis of your research and determines the type of knowledge you want to acquire (Parahoo, 2006). The following terms are associated with this step in the process – **paradigms** and **qualitative** and **quantitative approaches** (Mackenzie & Knipe, 2006). These terms and their definitions can be intertwined and can therefore be confusing to understand, however the following should address any confusion.

Key research paradigms are positivism, post-positivism, interpretivism, naturalism, constructivism, critical and postmodern (Grix, 2004; Blaxter *et al.*, 2006; Mackenzie & Knipe, 2006). The paradigms which appear to be used mostly in midwifery research are the positivist and naturalistic paradigms. They appear to be the two paradigms which hold the most opposing views. The **positivist paradigm** is considered to be the traditional paradigm underlying the scientific approach. This paradigm assumes that there is a fixed, orderly reality that can be objectively studied and is associated with quantitative research (Polit & Beck, 2008). The **naturalistic paradigm** is often considered to be an alternative paradigm to the positivist one. It maintains that there are multiple interpretations of reality and that the goal of research is to understand how individuals construct reality within their context. It is subjective and is associated with qualitative research (Letherby, 2003; Walsh & Wiggens, 2003).

The positivist research paradigm belongs to the scientific school of thought and its knowledge is usually derived in the form of randomised controlled trials (RCTs) and quasi-experiments (experimental research) and surveys in midwifery research. The naturalistic paradigm beliefs are focused on the human experience, thoughts and feelings and research is usually gathered using the research methods of ethnography, phenomenology, and grounded theory.

Qualitative and quantitative approaches can also be referred to as paradigms (Cluett & Bluff, 2006), but here, to aid your understanding, they are referred to as approaches. They help to structure the type of knowledge that needs to be acquired and different research methods are aligned to the different approaches, e.g. positivist paradigm, quantitative approach, randomised control trial or alternatively naturalistic paradigm, qualitative approach, ethnography.

In the **qualitative approach** the type of knowledge to be acquired focuses on experiences, thoughts, feelings and behaviour, and acknowledges the use of subjectivity (Davies, 2007). Its aim is to understand from the perspective of study participants, the meaning of their experiences (Robinson, 2002). An example of a qualitative study could be women's experiences of breastfeeding. The **quantitative approach** is centred within empirical knowledge, facts, figures, experiments, and is therefore tangible and objective (Begley, 2008). Its intention is to produce data that can be '*counted, measured, weighed, enumerated and so manipulated and compared mathematically*' (Grix, 2004, p. 173). An example of a quantitative study could be to measure the effectiveness of skin-to-skin contact on the length of breastfeeding.

Research language can be a bit overwhelming and to add to this further the student researcher must have an understanding of the following terms: epistemology, ontology, methodology, method and research design.

Epistemology is the study of the nature of knowledge, how we understand our world and relate this to the understanding of theories of what makes up

Table 1.1 Two possible research designs.

Paradigm	Approach	Methodology	Data collection tools	Data analysis
Naturalistic	Qualitative	Ethnography	Observation Field diaries Interviews	Thematic analysis
Positivist	Quantitative	Survey	Questionnaire	Descriptive statistics

knowledge (Cluett & Buff, 2006). It concerns *'questioning and understanding how we know what we know'* (Griffiths, 2009, p. 193). **Ontology** concerns *'our views about what constitutes the social world and how we can go about studying it'* (Barbour, 2008, p. 296). Walsh and Wiggens (2003, p. 3) suggest that *'ontological assumptions are the researcher's views about the nature of reality and epistemological assumptions are the researcher's decisions about how best to gather data on this reality'.*

In research texts there is quite often an intertwined use of the terms methodology and method, which can be confusing (Grix, 2004). To clarify, **methodology** refers to the theoretical and philosophical underpinnings of the research and the knowledge that is to be determined or theory developed (Barbour, 2008). **Method** comprises the procedural steps for data collection and data analysis (Brewer, 2000) and is the acquisition and analysis of that knowledge (Williams, 2008). Clark (2000, p. 46) suggests that clarity should be sought, when researchers are publishing their studies, regarding the use of the terms methodology and method as some researchers have failed to distinguish the difference between the research methodology (e.g. RCT, survey, ethnography) and the research methods used to collect and analyse the data (such as a questionnaire, a semi-structured interview or a rating scale). The methods selected are usually determined by the methodology chosen (Grix, 2004). The **research design** therefore encompasses all of the above, which is a detailed plan of the research study. Table 1.1 gives an outline of two research designs.

Audit and research

Audit and research share some similarities:

- Both involve answering specific questions which can relate to the quality of maternity care and practice.
- Both can be carried out either prospectively or retrospectively.
- Both involve some type of sampling, use of questionnaires for data collection and some form of analysis.
- Both have implications for midwifery practice.

Audit and research, however, involve different processes and work towards different goals.

What is audit?

A simple definition is that audit is a process of finding out whether systems or interventions that are evidence based are being carried out effectively.

The National Institute for Health & Clinical Excellence (NICE) describes clinical audit as:

> A quality improvement process that seeks to improve patient care and outcomes through systematic review of care against explicit criteria and the implementation of change. Aspects of the structure, processes and outcomes of care are selected and systematically evaluated against explicit criteria. Where indicated, changes are implemented at an individual, team, or service level and further monitoring is used to confirm improvement in healthcare delivery.
>
> Principles for Best Practice in Clinical Audit, NICE, 2002, p. 1

See Box 1.2.

The following ten statements clarify what audit is:

- Audit informs us if best practice is being carried out or not.
- Audit can identify systems failures and then make recommendations.
- Audit measures against set standards.
- Audit can measure the effects of a standardised treatment in use.
- Audit does not involve testing out new ideas, theories, treatments or interventions.
- Audit does not involve randomising service users to different treatment groups.
- Audit usually involves basic descriptive statistical analysis of data.
- Audit results are usually applicable to the local settings were the audit was carried out.
- Audit can also be undertaken nationally to compare systems and practices of local areas.
- Audit does not need ethical approval.

What is research?

'Research is the diligent, systematic inquiry or investigation to validate and refine existing knowledge and generate new knowledge' (Burns & Grove, 2009, p. 2). It can be defined further as the systematic collection of information to determine either an answer to a question, to test a theory or to verify a hunch (Lobiondo-Wood et al., 2002).

A simple definition is that research can involve investigating or exploring new ideas, theories or concepts, views and experiences, treatments or interventions to create new knowledge to inform education and promote best practice.

The following ten statements clarify what research is:

- Research creates new knowledge about what works and what is wanted by a target population.
- Research can make inferences about what will work for the population at large.
- Research can be based on a theory or hypothesis.

Box 1.2 An example of a clinical audit.

An acupuncturist midwife had an established clinic which provided pregnant women with the options of acupuncture, moxibustion and cupping therapies. In 2003, concerns about the evidence base and benefits of moxibustion led to it being suspended until a clinical audit was undertaken. Over an 18-month period a clinical audit was carried out by Calderdale and Huddersfield NHS Trust (2004). A review of the literature found that moxibustion reduced the need for External Cephalic Version (ECV), may be helpful to turn a breech presentation and no adverse effects were reported. Interestingly, during the audit period an increase in Caesarean Section (CS) for breech presentation when moxibustion therapy was discontinued prior to ECV being offered was reported. On the basis of this evidence permission was given to re-introduce this service for pregnant women.

Following this audit a Cochrane review has been carried out that examined the evidence investigating the effectiveness and safety of moxibustion on turning the baby from a breech position, the need for ECV, mode of birth and perinatal morbidity and mortality (Coyle *et al.*, 2005). The evidence supported the clinical audit outcomes. Three trials were included in this review with a total of 597 women. The reviewers were unable to undertake a meta-analysis of the data from the trials due to inconsistencies and differences within the trial methodologies and interventions. However, they reported that moxibustion reduced the need for ECV (RR 0.47, 95% CI 0.33–0.66) and decreased the use of oxytocin before or during labour for women who had vaginal deliveries (RR 0.28, 95% CI 0.13–0.60). They concluded that moxibustion may be helpful in turning a breech baby when applied to the little toe but there was insufficient evidence to support its use in clinical practice and recommended further research and well designed randomised controlled trials in moxibustion.

This NHS trust is now planning to undertake further research into the effectiveness of moxibustion.

- Research can involve investigating the effects of a treatment or interventions.
- Research may involve both descriptive and inferential statistical analysis of data.
- Research may involve emerging themes and concepts to generate new knowledge.
- Research can gain deep insights into understanding service users' feelings, views and experiences.
- Research requires ethics committee approval.
- Research can identify the gaps in knowledge that need further investigation or exploration.
- Research can provide the best evidence to promote good practices and standards.

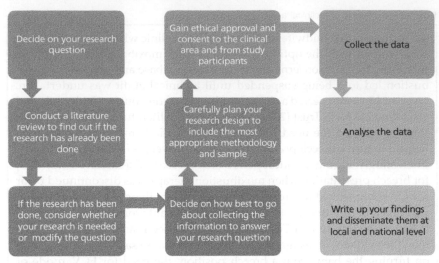

Figure 1.1 The research process.

Research–audit–audit–research cycle

Audit and research are intertwined. For research evidence to have an impact on maternity care and practice, audits have to be undertaken to monitor this. Research provides the evidence to promote best practice and enables the setting of standards to provide a high-quality service to women, their babies and families. Audit then plays an essential part and monitors the implementation of the evidence and seeks to find evidence that the standards are being carried out effectively and sufficiently. There is a research–audit–audit–research (RAAR) cycle, where research identifies areas for audit and then audit identifies areas for research.

Research process

A research study follows a structured process to access, collect and analyse information (Polit & Beck, 2006) and to verify the findings. Research can therefore be best described as a systematic process by which a question, a hunch or a theory can be identified, examined and analysed through a series of actions, in order to generate new knowledge or refine existing information. Figure 1.1 depicts the process of research as a series of actions.

According to Watson and Keady (2008), research can serve two purposes; these are to solve clinical problems and to fill gaps in knowledge. However, research really does not serve a purpose unless those findings are shared with others, which can be at local level with colleagues or to wider audiences such as publication in journals, and presentation at conferences. Research at its best can underpin good quality evidence-based practice which will be discussed later in this chapter.

The systematic approach adhered to throughout a research study will assist you to progress steadily (Box 1.3).

Box 1.3 Research process – ten points to remember.

---

* Define the subject and purpose.
* Study the research literature.
* Plan the research approach and methodology.
* Consider the ethical and governance aspects of the study.
* Carry out a pilot study.
* Collect the data.
* Analyse the data.
* Formulate conclusions.
* Discuss implications for midwifery practice.
* Disseminate (publication/conferences).

Research and Development Information (RDInfo)

The RDInfo website is an excellent resource for you to access as it provides excellent information on the research process and takes you through a step-by-step guide. The guide is clearly written and covers the systematic process of research which will help you methodically work through the different stages of the research process. For further information see http://www.RDInfo.

User involvement

It is considered good practice to involve women, their partners and family members, if applicable, in all stages of the research process. By doing so you will improve the quality of your research study as this will help you to gain an understanding from their perspective of what they deem to be important and necessary. This in turn should then increase the likelihood of you completing your research successfully as you have listened to their views and what they feel will make a difference to their care or involvement.

RDInfo suggests that you can distinctly involve service users in four stages of the research process:

* Setting the research agenda.
* Developing the proposal.
* During the conduct of the project.
* Disseminating results.

Setting the research agenda

Involve users in decision making and consider what is important to them and not just of academic or research interest to you.

Developing the proposal

Involving people who may participate in your research or who have an interest in this area will help you to design a more pragmatic study with a higher rate of success.

During the conduct of the project

Check things out and ask service users and participants as this will help you identify any potential problems that may arise and give you an insight into how you can address these and make improvements. This will help you to complete your study successfully and on time.

Disseminating results

Remember to disseminate your results widely and not just to the professionals; you should include users as this will help you bridge the theory–practice gap. It is interesting to note that funding bodies now require evidence of, firstly, how users have been consulted and involved in the designing of a research proposal, secondly, how they have contributed to the undertaking of the research study and, thirdly, how they are going to be involved in your dissemination plan.

INVOLVE

In the UK, INVOLVE is a well established national advisory group of about 20 members involving users, researchers and representatives from the public and voluntary sector. INVOLVE was set up in 1996 and is funded by the Department of Health. INVOLVE aims to promote and support active user involvement in research that is carried out by NHS, public health and social care services.

The chief executive of the Terence Higgins Trust and chair of INVOLVE, Nick Partridge, states on their website, *'When the public get involved in research it becomes more relevant to people's needs, more reliable and more likely to be used.'*

This group has produced several publications to guide researchers, users and funding organisations, has a mailing list and provides a quarterly newsletter. For further information see INVOLVE'S website http://www.invo.org.uk/.

Service development projects

Service development projects are often used to implement good practice and will involve some form of evaluation of the initiative. Again, you need to consider user involvement. However, if your project is not considered to be research then you do not need ethical approval but will need to consider good practice and clinical governance aspects.

Box 1.4 is an example of a successful midwifery-led service development project (Steen, 2007).

Introducing qualitative research

Qualitative research involves exploring opinions, behaviours and experiences from the participants' points of view, thereby determining what something means from the perspectives of those taking part in the research study. Subjectivity is integral to the researcher's role in this approach as it allows for better understanding of the subject under investigation by the researcher (Robinson, 2002).

Box 1.4   The Maternal Health & Well-Being Project.

Background: The Department of Health has acknowledged that 'Healthy mothers are key for giving healthy babies a healthy start in life' (Department of Health, 2004).

Service development project: A health and fitness initiative for mums-to-be and new mums was developed in collaboration with the maternity services of a large NHS trust and the health and leisure services of a local authority. Following a successful pilot study, approval to continue and evaluate the initiative for a 1-year period was given.

The aim: To promote health and fitness during pregnancy, prepare for birth and then maintain health and fitness after childbirth.

The initiative: Women attended a rolling on programme of 6 antenatal workshop/exercise classes from 16 weeks gestation. These women then returned to the postnatal workshop/exercise classes 2 weeks after birth with their newborn baby. A midwife and fitness instructor at a local sports centre ran the sessions. 'Prescription for Activity' passes were then offered to women on completion of the programme to encourage them to continue to exercise for a further 12 weeks and attend mainstream classes and the gym.

Findings: Health and well-being benefits were reported on evaluation of the workshops and exercise classes. Women appear to have enjoyed exercising in a friendly environment, with adequate facilities and at an affordable cost. A majority of women continued to exercise and many of their partners also began to exercise. See poster below and www.bbc.co.uk/leeds/features/living/fitness/pregnancy_pilates.shtml.

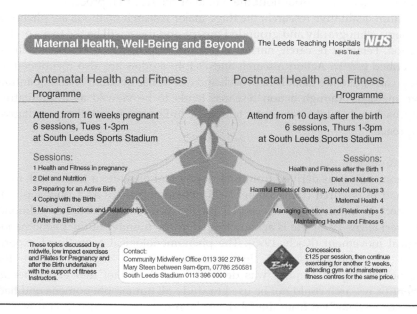

Box 1.5 Characteristics of the qualitative approach.

---

* Inductive.
* Explores – thoughts, feelings, experiences, beliefs and social interactions.
* Describes and interprets.
* Sampling is usually purposive, but convenience, snowballing, open and theoretical can also be utilised.
* Information can be collected by observation, interviews and visual analysis of documents or objects.
* Analysis of the data – usually thematic analysis and more specific analysis for phenomenology and grounded theory.
* Subjective.
* Not generalisable.

Some researchers may consider it to be an easier option than quantitative research, but having conducted both qualitative and quantitative studies, we know it is not. It can be very time consuming, but the experience and sense of satisfaction in producing research whose whole basis is the participants' experience is very rewarding (Mapp & Hudson, 2005). Box 1.5 describes the characteristics of the qualitative approach.

Reflexivity is integral to qualitative research. It involves researchers acknowledging their personal biases, therefore being self-aware. It can ensure trustworthiness of research findings (Kingdon, 2005). It is a process that should be ongoing throughout the whole of the research process.

Within qualitative research, the three major research methods are phenomenology, ethnography and grounded theory, and these will be the focus of this section. Feminist research, narrative research and historical research will be described briefly. Action research and Delphi studies are also mentioned as they can both use a flexible approach and can utilise qualitative and quantitative methods, though action research tends to be viewed as a qualitative approach and Delphi techniques tend to be linked more with the quantitative approach.

Phenomenology

Phenomenology is derived from philosophy and provides a framework for a method of research (Denscombe, 2003). Phenomenology as a philosophical method of inquiry was developed by the German philosopher Edmond Husserl (1859–1938). He is acknowledged as the founder of the phenomenological movement (Koch, 1995). The phenomenological term 'lived experience' is synonymous with this research approach. Husserl's drive for phenomenological enquiry was derived from the belief that experimental scientific research could not be used to study all human phenomena and had become so detached from the fabric of the human experience, that it was in fact obstructing our understanding of ourselves (Crotty, 1996). He felt driven to establish a rigorous science that found truth in the lived experience (LoBiondo-Wood & Haber, 2002).

The goal of Husserlian phenomenological enquiry is to fully describe a lived experience and to develop insights from the perspectives of those involved, by them detailing their lived experience of a particular time in their lives (Clark, 2000). It stresses that only those that have experienced phenomena can communicate them to the outside world (Todres & Holloway, 2004). It therefore answers questions of meaning, in understanding an experience from those who have experienced it (Mapp, 2008).

Husserlian phenomenology is about searching for meanings and essences of the experience, and advocates 'bracketing', which is the suspension of the researcher's own preconceptions, beliefs or prejudices so that they do not influence the description of the respondents' experience (Parahoo, 2006). It obtains descriptions of experiences through first-person accounts during informal one-to-one interviews. These are then transcribed and analysed for themes and meanings (Moustakas, 1994), allowing the experience to be understood.

Although Husserl founded the phenomenological approach (Polit et al., 2001), it is not the single phenomenological method. Other phenomenologists who have shaped this approach are Gabriel Marcel (1889–1973), Jean-Paul Sartre (1905–1980) and Maurice Merleau-Ponty (1908–1961). According to Cohen (2000) they are referred to as the French phase of phenomenology, whereas Husserl and Martin Heidegger (who was mentored by the former) are the German phase.

Heidegger developed another phenomenological approach known as 'hermeneutics', meaning interpretation (Annells, 1996). It differs from Husserlian phenomenology, in that the researchers bring their own understanding and experiences to the research process, whereas the former advocates bracketing (Walters, 1995). Husserlian phenomenology therefore requires the researcher to suspend personal beliefs about the research phenomena, whilst seeking to describe the participants' experiences. Conversely, Heideggerian phenomenology suggests that researchers interpret the data collected in terms of their own personal experiences (Mapp, 2008).

There are three schools of phenomenology (Polit et al., 2001), and the first two are the focus for midwifery and nursing research (Mapp, 2008). The first school follows the Husserlian approach; its main focus is on description. The second school is guided by the Heideggerian approach, utilising interpretive hermeneutics as its basis. The third school is referred to as the Dutch or Utrecht school, its approach combines the characteristics of descriptive and interpretive phenomenology (Holloway & Wheeler, 2002).

> Phenomenology has different applications dependent on the authors who have founded and developed it. This should therefore be recognized in midwifery research to increase knowledge and the use of the most appropriate phenomenological research approach for the phenomenon to be studied. Following a Husserlian approach the researcher will aim to 'bracket' her beliefs to describe

Box 1.6 An example of a midwifery Husserlian phenomenology study.

Feelings and fears during obstetric emergencies Part 1 (Mapp & Hudson, 2005).

This study was of a purposive sample of ten women who detailed their lived experiences of an obstetric emergency. Data collection was unstructured one-to-one interviews. Colaizzi's method of data analysis was utilised.

the experience people have had, as opposed to using a Heiderggerian approach, whereby the experiences are interpreted and analysed through the researcher's own knowledge and experience.

Mapp, 2008, p. 309

An example of a Husserlian study is given in Box 1.6.

As phenomenology requires the exploration of the whole person, it is deemed to be particularly suitable in studying phenomena relative to midwifery. It enables midwives to study in depth the childbirth process directly in context with those who are experiencing it. In particular it facilitates a woman's unique experience of childbirth which would otherwise be unknown, and which can potentially assist improvements in practice (Mapp, 2008).

Ethnography

Ethnography can be defined as *'a qualitative research approach developed by anthropologists with the purpose of describing an aspect of culture, but is also aimed at learning about the culture or factor being studied'* (Lanoe, 2002, p. 94). It is considered to be the oldest of the qualitative research methodologies. It has been in use since ancient times, the Greeks and the Romans wrote descriptions of cultures they encountered. The term ethnography is derived from Greek and it means a description of people (Holloway & Wheeler, 2002). Ethnography as a research design aims to be holistic by studying *'naturally occurring human behaviour through observation'* (Brink & Edgecombe, 2003, p. 1028).

Ethnography has its roots in anthropology, but it is becoming increasingly popular in the field of healthcare research to study behaviour and social interactions, and specifically in midwifery, to explore the culture of childbirth (Clark, 2000). Anthropologists use ethnography to produce knowledge, whereas health researchers aim to produce knowledge to improve practice (Holloway & Wheeler, 2002). Ethnography appears, therefore, to be well suited to healthcare research, whereby the researchers are not just describing behaviour, but are aiming to make sense of it with the potential for making improvements in practice (Holloway & Todres, 2006).

Ethnography came to public attention in the 1920s with the advent of anthropologists studying ancient tribes and cultures, pith-helmeted explorers expounded by the works of Malinowski (1922) and Mead (1943) (cited by

Box 1.7 An example of an ethnographic midwifery study.

> *An ethnography of experienced midwives caring for women in labour* (Price & Johnson, 2006).
>
> This study used a purposive sample of six midwives. Data collection included participant observation, to study encounters between midwives and the women in their care, and semi-structured interviews. The interviews were felt to be a vital component to the research process to confirm the researchers' interpretations of the behaviour observed. Thematic analysis was used to analyse the data.

Box 1.8 Types of ethnography (Roberts, 2009, p. 292).

> - Classical ethnography – prolonged contact with a group, which is studied.
> - Systematic ethnography – attempts to define and delineate a specific cultural structure.
> - Interpretive ethnography – attempts to discover the meanings of social interaction and behaviour (Donovan, 2006, p. 174).
> - Descriptive ethnography – describes what is happening.
> - Critical ethnography – emphasises the subjectivity of the researcher and focuses on power interactions (Holloway & Todres, 2006).

Denscombe, 2003). Ethnography did not find its roots in applied midwifery research until the late 1980s and since then it has gained in popularity and has been used to explore the culture of childbirth and the education of student midwives (Davies, 1996; John & Parsons, 2006; Price & Johnson, 2006). The two pivotal midwifery ethnographic studies which are considered to have given credence to ethnography as a research methodology, were Mavis Kirkham's (1987) PhD, *Basic supportive care in labour: interaction with women and around women in labour* (cited by Donovan, 2006) and Sheila Hunt's study of two labour wards, published in *The Social Meaning of Midwifery* (Hunt & Symonds, 1995). See Box 1.7.

The focus of ethnography is on *'individuals, not in isolation, but in relation to their organisations, communities, customs and culture'* (Clark, 2000, p. 44). It is a research methodology (Lindsay, 2007) that can enable researchers to make sense of people's actions by observing them in the context of their environment, (Varcoe *et al.*, 2003). This then allows for an understanding of their behaviour within their cultural arena, such as midwives working on a labour ward. This demonstrates the whole essence of ethnography, which allows for the researcher to become immersed within the culture to gain an understanding of the behaviour for that particular group of people. It must be stressed, however, that within ethnography there are different types (Roberts, 2009) and Box 1.8 gives an outline of the various characteristics.

Grounded theory

Grounded theory focuses on generating a theory from research data, to describe and explain what is happening in a social setting or interaction (Rees, 2003). The researcher has an area of research interest and is then led by the research data (Parahoo, 2006). This is in contrast to other research methodologies, when the purpose is either to test a hypothesis or answer a question at the start of the research process (Davies, 2007).

Grounded theory as a research methodology was discovered by social scientists Barney Glaser & Anselm Strauss in 1967. Their book *The Discovery of Grounded Theory* (Glaser & Strauss, 1967) was their only publication together on the subject. Since then they have published separately on this topic, with apparent similar conceptual ideologies, but differing applications (Strauss & Corbin 1997; Glaser, 1998; Strauss & Corbin, 1998; Glaser, 2001).

Symbolic interactionism is a key feature of grounded theory (Polit & Beck, 2006, p. 222), *'which focuses on the manner in which people make sense of social interactions and the interpretations they attach to social symbols e.g. language'*. Grounded theory therefore seeks to identify and explain what is happening in a social setting (Roberts, 2008). It aims to be true to the reality of the situation/interaction under investigation (Letherby, 2003) and is being increasingly used in healthcare research (Dykes, 2004).

Grounded theory can be used within both the quantitative and qualitative approaches (Boychuk Duchscher & Morgan, 2004). However, it is most commonly found in the latter, due to the flexibility that is required of its research design (Bluff, 2006). It differs from other research methodologies in that a literature review is not usually conducted until the conclusion of the study, so that the research is conducted without any preconceived theories, therefore allowing ideas to develop (Grix, 2004). Grounded theory also differs in that data collection and data analysis proceed in parallel from the beginning of the study and interact continuously to allow the data to lead the researcher in developing new theories (Strauss & Corbin, 1998).

Grounded theory is a research methodology that can provide a framework for midwifery researchers to produce interesting and innovative research. It can start with an area of interest, with the researchers being open to being led wherever the data will take them, thus providing new perspectives on midwifery care (Roberts, 2008). Box 1.9 gives an example of a midwifery grounded theory study.

Feminist research

Feminist research is not just research on women conducted by women; it is much more complex than that. It is about recognising oppression and the reasons for it, valuing women's experiences and understanding the actions that can be taken to change the situation (Kralik & van Loon, 2008). Feminist research studies *'are based on women making sense of their own lives and facilitating collective action to change their social situation'*. Therefore an objective of this research perspective is to create change and not just the creation of knowledge (Kralik & van Loon, 2008, p. 42). Feminism is the 'theoretical perspective' and

Box 1.9 An example of a midwifery grounded theory study.

Breaking the rules in baby-feeding practice in the UK: deviance and good practice? (Furber & Thomson, 2006).

This study used theoretical sampling and 30 midwives volunteered to participate. Data collection was semi-structured interviews and field notes completed at the conclusion of the interview. Data analysis used was specific to grounded theory, constant comparative analysis method.

Box 1.10 An example of a midwifery feminist study.

The practice setting: site of ethical conflict for some mothers and midwives (Thompson, 2003).

This study was conducted from a feminist perspective. Snowball sampling was used; eight childbearing women and eight midwives participated. Data collection involved the personal narratives of mothers and midwives about what they considered to be ethical conflicts. Data analysis was guided by feminist ethics and the participants and researcher jointly analysed and interpreted the data for emerging themes (thematic analysis).

encompassed within this are many different 'schools' of feminism. If the researcher has therefore decided to conduct a feminist study, she then must consider the feminist perspective that she will follow and the most appropriate research methodology that matches the study's aims (Dykes, 2004). Box 1.10 gives an example of a midwifery feminist study.

Historical research

Historical research is about examining events in the past that are related to midwifery practice. It can enable greater understanding of the midwifery profession. More recently, this type of research has moved to become 'interpretive history', this means to try and search for meanings and therefore understanding of events in the past from the viewpoint of the present (Burns & Grove, 2009). Information can be collected from many different sources: books, journals, documentaries, films, newspapers, written narratives, diaries, songs, interviews (oral histories), etc. Therefore, the data collected will be realised in a textual format, e.g. written words that will require analysis. Analysis within this context can take different forms depending on the type of text presented, e.g. discourse analysis or textual analysis. Discourse analysis (Rugg & Petrie, 2007) would be appropriate for dialogue or conversations, whereas textual analysis may be appropriate for newspaper coverage (McKee, 2003). Engaging in historical research can be a time consuming process that needs to be systematic and rigorous in its approach and application (Fealy,

Box 1.11 An example of a midwifery historical study.

> *Using oral history in midwifery* (Reid, 2004).
>
> This article describes a study that gained oral accounts of the history of Scottish midwives in the twentieth century. Snowball sampling was used. Forty-five midwives took part, ranging in qualification dates from 1928 to 1981. Data collection, included interview narratives – the participants 'told their stories'; however, some open questions were also used to guide the interview (interview guide used). Data collection produced a rich description of midwifery history. Data analysis produced specific oral testimonies on certain issues highlighted in the transcriptions (thematic analysis).

Box 1.12 An example of a midwifery narrative study.

> *Why women choose midwifery: a narrative analysis of motivations and understandings in a group of first-year student midwives* (Williams, 2006).
>
> The study included a self-selected sample of 15 first-year student midwives. Data collection was individual interviews – narrative approach with an interview guide. Data analysis was done by narrative analysis (thematic analysis).

2008), yet it can produce very interesting and worthwhile information. Box 1.11 gives an example of a midwifery historical study.

Narrative research
Narrative research is essentially the collection and analysis of stories. In the last decade it has developed into an accepted approach in qualitative studies (Hurtwitz *et al.*, 2004) and become popular in health research (Griffiths, 2009). '*A story narrative is a personal account of a sequence of actions or events, told to another person (or written for a reader)*'. Narrative research is not just about someone describing events, but it is about how they have made sense/ understood what happened and how it made them feel (Greenhalgh & Wengraf, 2008, p. 244). Narrative '*analysis seeks meaning and purpose in the telling of the story*' (Griffiths, 2009, p. 196). Data analysis utilised for this approach would be thematic analysis. Box 1.12 gives an example of a midwifery narrative study.

Action research (flexible approach)
The focus on change is key to the action research process. Action research was developed by Kurt Lewins in the 1940s to resolve social conflicts. '*The primary purpose of action-based research is to bring about change in specific situations, in local systems and real-world environments with aims to solve real problems*' (Parkin, 2009, p. 20).

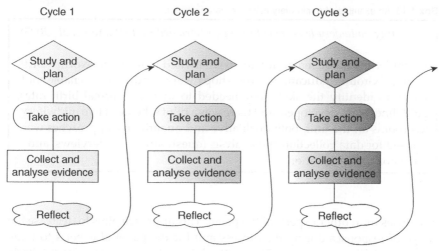

Figure 1.2 Progressive problem solving with action research. Source: http://cadres.pepperdine. edu/ccar/define.html. Reproduced with permission from Dr Margaret Riel.

Action researchers are part of the situation and together with practitioners in the clinical area, they identify a problem, initiate change, gather the evidence to assess the effectiveness of the change, make further refinements and assessments until an improvement/benefit is demonstrated (Waterman & Hope, 2008). This process is referred to as the action research cycle or flexible spiral process (Blaxter *et al.*, 2006). Figure 1.2 is a depiction of this process (Reil, 2007).

Action research can be broadly assigned to two types. The first is where an expert researcher leads the process with the involvement of the practitioners being studied (action research). Secondly, there is participatory action research, where the process is led by the practitioners and the distinction between (expert) researcher and practitioner is removed, however the practitioners can ask for advice from the researcher without rescinding control (Lindsay, 2007). Data collection can include both qualitative and quantitative methods (Polit & Beck, 2008). See Box 1.13 for an example of a midwifery action research study.

Delphi study (flexible approach)

A Delphi study may be seen as a structured process within which qualitative, quantitative or mixed methods can be used to promote an interactive forecasting approach which relies on a panel of independent experts (Skulmoski *et al.*, 2007). These experts complete questionnaires in two or more rounds. After each round, a researcher provides an anonymous summary of the combined experts' answers or what are often referred to as forecasts (estimations) from the previous round and the reasons given to support their judgements. The experts are then encouraged to revise their earlier answers in light of the

Box 1.13 An example of a midwifery action research project.

Promoting midwifery-led care within an obstetric-led unit (Walton *et al.*, 2005).

All midwives at the maternity unit were invited to form the 'Normal Birth Strategy Group'. Educational workshops were conducted to enable midwives to identify the skills they needed to increase normal birth rates, guidelines were developed, and there was a pilot scheme of two midwifery-led rooms on the unit. Both qualitative and quantitative approaches were utilised for data collection and analysis (questionnaires, interviews, audit, reflection and evaluation).

---

responses from other experts of the panel. This approach aims to decrease the range of responses during the process and for the panel of experts to unite towards similar responses. The methodology has predetermined criteria which indicate when to stop collecting data, such as the number of rounds, when a level of consensus has been reached and the findings are consistent. Average scores and the mean or median are scoring high levels of agreement. The Delphi method is based on the assumption that group judgements are more credible than individual judgements.

> A process of developing ideas and forming a consensus about an issue among a group of people without them being in contact with each other.
>
> Griffiths, 2009, p. 192

The group of people is referred to as a panel of experts on the topic of the research question (Hasson *et al.*, 2000). The information can be gathered by post, face-to-face panels and more popularly by e-mail; the questions posed to the experts are usually collated in a questionnaire. The researcher identifies the level of consensus among the experts' responses and the original, and combined analysed answers are returned to the panel for them to further rank/rate them. This process of returning the analysed responses to the panel can happen many times until the researcher determines that a consensus has been reached (Walsh & Wiggens, 2003). As to the size of the sample (panel of experts), there appears no clear guidance, however McKenna and Keeney (2008) would suggest that a small group of interested experts would achieve a good response rate and therefore reach a consensus, rather than a large group whose response may be poor. See Box 1.14.

Introducing quantitative research

Quantitative research is a general term used to describe research that aims to measure concepts or events as objectively as is feasibly possible by numerical and statistical means.

Box 1.14 An example of a midwifery Delphi study.

Registration requirements for midwives in Australia: a Delphi study (Pincombe *et al.*, 2007).

The sample consisted of a panel of 36 experts. They were invited to participate by a letter, the aim being to gain a consensus on the minimum requirements for midwifery registration. Data collection involved three rounds of postal questionnaires which included both qualitative and quantitative questions for the panel to reach a consensus. Data analysis used thematic content analysis and descriptive statistics.

It is important from the outset that you are able to distinguish between what a quantitative research approach is and what quantitative methods and studies are available for you to use. Generally speaking, a research approach describes the whole design of the research study; this includes its philosophical stance, i.e. positivism, the methodology, type of data to be collected and analysed and how the results will be presented. This approach is often referred to as being reductionist, deterministic or deductive in its approach (Parahoo, 2006). It can involve measuring how variables interact (cause and effect) and also make comparisons and find correlations.

A quantitative approach involves stating a research question or a hypothesis and then designing the study to collect data to undertake some sort of numerical analysis to answer the research question or provide evidence to confirm or refute a hypothesis. A quantitative method is used when there is a need to provide accurate and precise measurements such as facts and figures to help us understand an issue and how to resolve it. Remember the whole process should reflect objectivity and provide valid and reliable results. However, realistically this is not as straightforward as it initially appears and all research, whether it uses a quantitative or qualitative approach, will have limitations and biases that need to be considered. A researcher must consider how to minimise the limitations and biases as far as possible when designing the study. Quantitative research will use a measurement where numbers can be genuinely real numbers such as maternal age or a baby's birth weight or be assigned to represent people, objects, events, attitudes and levels of severity, intensity or agreement. To promote objectivity data collection tools such as structured questionnaires and structured interviews are used to collect the data; sampling methods such as random sampling and sample size are also used and estimated to further promote objectivity. See Chapter 6.

Data are analysed in numbers (often referred to as 'number crunching') and will describe the distribution in a population and determine whether there are any relationships between variables measured to understand the phenomena being investigated. Often a researcher will construct or use valid numerical or rating scales to help measure and interpret the data. Once the numerical data have been analysed they have to be described and discussed; graphs and charts are helpful to interpret the findings visually. Data terms such as frequencies, proportions, percentages, amounts, prevalence, incidences, trends and patterns are associated with quantitative research.

Quantitative research studies

There are several types of quantitative research studies that can be non-experimental (descriptive or observational) or experimental (true experiments or comparative studies) in their approach and can be used to find evidence to inform clinical practice, test a treatment or intervention and indicate the need for further research that may involve different research approaches.

Non-experimental design
Case studies

Case studies can involve a participant or participants who already have a social habit, condition or illness and are compared with participant(s) who do not.

For example: a study on pregnant women who continue to smoke during pregnancy; they are asked their reasons why and the answers are then compared with a sample of women who have stopped smoking during pregnancy.

The main advantages of case studies are:

- They can be carried out relatively quickly.
- Asking pregnant women about their reasons for doing something, e.g. smoking, will help a researcher to find out quickly some answers that otherwise could take a lot longer to ascertain with other research methods.
- The research method is straightforward and a researcher does not need a control group or to randomly allocate women.
- Women are simply approached at booking to participate and if consent is given are then asked a few questions.

Case studies, however, provide limited evidence and there is potential bias concerning recall and selection. The studies are not generalisible to the population at large but can be undertaken prior to a cohort study or randomised controlled study to indicate the need for further research.

Case series

Case series and case reports can consist of either a collection of records/reports on conditions and treatments or therapies that an individual woman receives, or of records/reports on a single woman.

For example: at an antenatal booking appointment a woman presents with a rare condition that you have never heard of before and you need to find information and guidance on how to care for her. A search for case series or case records/reports may reveal information and guidance that will assist you to plan her care. Case series and case record/reports use no control groups with which to compare outcomes and therefore provide limited evidence.

Box 1.15 Example of a midwifery cohort study.

Dahlen *et al.* (2007) carried out a prospective cohort study of risk factors for severe perineal trauma (third- and fourth-degree tears) during childbirth over a 2-year period. A hospital's computerised obstetric information system was used and midwives were asked to comment on possible reasons for severe perineal trauma. Data were prospectively gathered on 6595 women who gave birth from 1 April, 1998 to 31 March, 2000 and analysed following the exclusion of women who had either an emergency or elective Caesarean section. The primary outcome was the presence or absence of severe perineal trauma for identified risk factors. The overall incidence of severe perineal trauma involved 134 (2%) of women. Of these women 122 (91%) had third-degree tears and 12 (9%) had fourth-degree tears. Primiparity, instrumental delivery, Asian ethnicity and large babies were associated with an elevated risk of severe perineal trauma and the researchers concluded that these findings confirm current knowledge. Lack of effective communication with the woman during the birth, different birth positions, delivery technique, ethnicity and obstetric influences were suggested by midwives as some reasons for the incidence of severe perineal trauma.

Cohort studies
A cohort study can involve a group of participants who have a condition or receive a particular treatment/intervention and are followed up over a long period of time and compared with a group who do not have the condition or receive the treatment/intervention under investigation.

For example: a follow-up study would compare the group of women who continued to smoke during pregnancy with the group who did not and monitor any health problems they develop over time. Cohort studies are not as reliable as randomised controlled studies, since the two groups may differ and random allocation and confounding variables are not controlled for.

The main disadvantage with cohort studies is the duration of time. Many changes (social, physical and/or environmental) can occur during the study follow-up period. For example, women can move away, have other children, divorce, remarry, develop illnesses, receive treatments, and even die. See Box 1.15.

Prospective studies
Prospective studies look at data that are going to be generated, the events having not yet occurred. A midwifery example that challenged evidence reported by Friedman (1954), who developed what are known as the 'Friedman Curves' of labour (based on a sample of only 100 women and some of the sample had oxytocin augmentation of their labours), has made an impact on how we assess and interpret the length of labour. See Box 1.16.

Box 1.16 How long is normal labour?

Albers *et al.* (1996) and Albers (1999) assessed the length of first and second stages of labour in two studies. Women who had a normal birth (at term, spontaneous onset of labour, cephalic presentation, singleton, no medical problems and no induction or augmentation of labour or epidural) were included and descriptive data were measured. These studies found that women who had a first stage with a normal limit was twice that found by Friedman but length of second stage was similar:

Primigravidae: First stage 19.4/17.5/8.5   Second stage 147/147/150
(hour)   (minute)
Multigravidae: First stage 13.7/13.8/7.0   Second stage 57/64/60
(hour)   (minute)

Basically, this indicated that the normal progress in the first stage of labour in the samples studied was on average 0.5 cm an hour of cervical dilation, which was less than half the rate that Friedman found (1 cm).

Retrospective studies
Retrospective studies look at recorded data that can be gathered from several written sources such as case notes, case studies, clinical reports, policies, guidelines and media material. The evidence can be analysed and comparisons can be made.

An example: a retrospective study undertaken by Nixon *et al.* (1998) compared outcomes of term infants of average birth weight with outcomes of large infants in a nurse-midwifery service. Data were retrieved from a computer data base that contained information from a data form routinely completed for all births. The study population included 2228, of which 322 (14.5%) of the infants weighed 4000 g or more. These large infants had birth outcomes comparable with those reported by others in the medical literature, suggesting that nurse-midwifery management, including consultation with physician colleagues, can be appropriate and safe.

Surveys
Survey methodology is a well known quantitative research method and aims to collect large amounts of data about a specific target population (population of interest). A survey is the most common questionnaire method used to describe social phenomena and has its origins in Victorian Britain (Bowling, 2009). Descriptive data describing populations and their attributes, such as level of knowledge, skills, views, attitudes, behaviours, incidences etc., can be recorded and inferences can be made to the total population. Researchers look for associations between variables and then patterns and trends. Government surveys are a good example of this methodology and these give information about national trends and issues. See Box 1.17.

Box 1.17 British Crime Survey (BCS) (2010).

The British Crime Survey (BCS) is an annual national survey that reports information gathered from face-to-face interviews of a sample of the general population residing in households in England and Wales. This information is combined with police recorded crime data that estimates the amount of crime in England and Wales.

The most recent *British Crime Survey*, reported by the Home Office (July 2010), involved 44 638 face-to-face interviews. This survey reported that men were twice as likely as women (4.2% compared with 1.8%) to have experienced violence in the year prior to the interview. Domestic violence accounted for 14% of all violent incidents and there was no change in the proportion of men or women experiencing domestic violence. Women were at greater risk than men of experiencing domestic violence (0.4% compared with 0.2%). Seven percent of women (16–59 years) compared with 4% of men (16–59 years) experienced domestic violence in the year prior to interview. This survey has implications for the health sector in general and within maternity services. Preventing future cases of domestic violence will reduce both maternal and fetal mortality and morbidity rates, yet there is limited research to demonstrate effective preventative measures. Presently, midwifery-led research within this neglected area is ongoing (Steen-Greaves *et al.*, 2009) and could form the foundations for further research in this field.

Generally postal surveys are used with the inclusion of a stamped addressed envelope to encourage respondents to return the completed questionnaire, but telephone or face-to-face approaches are an alternative way to collect structured/semi-structured information. However, the internet has impacted on how surveys are conducted and on-line surveys are becoming more popular as they appear to be a faster and an easier method to collect data and for respondents to complete.

When undertaking a survey it is the researcher's responsibility to clearly define the target population and ensure a representative sample is recruited to be able to analyse the data and make inferences to the population at large. See Chapter 6, Basic Statistics section.

For example: a typical target population could be all pregnant women booked between January 2009 and December 2010 who are classified as high risk. Randomly selected consultant-led maternity units representing the four countries of the UK could be used to recruit a representative sample size from which inferences could be made to all consultant-led maternity units in the UK.

Surveys are helpful to ask the 'what', 'where', 'when' and 'how' but not as helpful to ask the 'why' types of questions (Bell, 2005). Surveys can establish associations but not causality and are susceptible to recall bias. See Box 1.18.

Box 1.18 A midwifery example of a survey undertaken by Lavender *et al.* (2005).

A postal survey conducted in England in January 2003 to May 2004 explored the views of consultant obstetricians and heads of midwifery on women's requests for Caesarean section without clinical indication and of a possible randomised controlled trial. Semi-structured questionnaires with closed and open questions were used to collect data and make comparisons between the two professional groups. Chi-square test was used to compare the proportion of respondents saying 'yes' to each question and open responses were analysed manually. A good response rate was reported, 660/924 (71%) eligible obstetricians and 123/169 (73%) midwives responded. Almost half of the obstetricians and a quarter of midwives believed that a woman should choose her method of delivery. A minority thought a trial was feasible, ethical, or desirable. Female obstetricians were less likely to support a trial than male ones. Whether or not the obstetrician and midwife had children did not influence their responses; nor did the type of unit in which the professionals worked.

Experimental design
Comparative studies
Comparative studies are studies where a planned treatment/intervention is given to a group of participants to assess its effect and compare this with a group that has not had the treatment/intervention. A comparative study where random allocation is not carried out is referred to as a quasi-experimental design.

An **historical example:** *Treatise of Scurvy* (Lind, 1753). In the eighteenth century James Lind spent 6 years studying scurvy in sailors aboard HMS Salisbury. He provided some sailors (not all) with a diet that included fruit and vegetables and then observed the results and concluded those in the 'intervention group' (fruit and vegetables) were more likely to remain free of scurvy. See web link for further information: http://www.jameslindlibrary.org/trial_records/17th_18th_Century/lind/lind_tp.html.

It is important to note that participants are not randomly assigned to a treatment/intervention group or comparison group(s). Some recruitment selection method, however, can be used such as, alternate days of the week, admission to a postnatal ward etc. This can introduce selection bias as the target population are not given an equal opportunity to be recruited to the study. See Box 1.19.

Pragmatic studies
Evidence-based guidelines and policies have encouraged the undertaking of pragmatic studies. A pragmatic trial is designed to measure whether an intervention/treatment is effective when used in usual circumstances. Participants should be representative of the target population to whom the

Box 1.19 A midwifery example of a comparative study (quasi-experimental design).

Barclay and Martin (1983) carried out a study which investigated the effectiveness of 'witch hazel', 'a no localised treatment', 'iced sitz bath', 'warm sitz bath', 'ray lamp' groups. Treatments were given three to four times daily for 10 minutes during the first 5 days following suturing of an episiotomy. Outcomes of pain, healing and infection rates were assessed from day 1 to day 5. Analgesia use was assessed and then classified as regular users if the woman had medication 4-hourly to 8-hourly for 24 hours or more. The researchers used a five-point verbal rating scale to assess the severity of pain and devised their own five-point ordinal scales to assess healing and signs of infection. The researchers reported that they would not be introducing the use of witch hazel as a means to alleviate perineal pain as it proved to be less beneficial on both subjective and objective measures when compared with iced sitz baths and no treatment.

intervention/treatment will be given in a real world setting if effectiveness is found. The participants maybe randomised or non-randomised.

Pre and post comparative studies
Data are collected before and then after a treatment/intervention is given to an experimental group. This type of study can involve one or more groups and comparisons are made. Sometimes, pre and post comparative studies are referred to as a time series study as participants are retested over a period of time. Ideally a researcher will take a set of baseline observations/tests before giving the treatment/intervention. Post observations/tests will also be measured over a period of time following the treatment/intervention being given to see if it makes a difference to the participants. This type of study is often used for service evaluation. See Box 1.20 for an example of a service evaluation pre and post comparative study.

Crossover trials
A crossover trial is a controlled trial where each participant, selected through a clear inclusion criteria, receives both the control and treatment/intervention in a random order, i.e. randomised to control group (A) then (crossover) and commence treatment/intervention group (B) and paired comparisons can be made.
    The main advantages are:

• All participants are their own controls and this reduces the sample size.
• All participants receive treatment/intervention and blinding can happen.
• Statistical analysis can be undertaken and comparisons can be made.
• Participants may feel more willing to participate as they have an opportunity to try both treatments.

Box 1.20 An example of a service evaluation pre and post comparative study in New Zealand.

The nursing and midwifery clinical handover project compared pre and post-test data. This project involved staff and patients from three wards (one being a postnatal ward) at Waikato Hospital, New Zealand (Wynne-Jones, 2008). Pre-test involved investigating and exploring current practice of nursing/midwifery shift handover. Staff and patient feedback gave baseline data and there was evidence that the duration of handover and duplication of information was a common problem. Other factors were identified such as staff disruptive behaviour, poor punctuality, where and how the handover was carried out, i.e. office setting, at the bedside, by a coordinator to all staff, or one-to-one handovers. A new standardised process was implemented (succinct global handovers followed by bedside handover involving the patient and a checklist with reference to documentation). Post-test results demonstrated that most patients and staff supported bedside handovers but some concerns were raised with regards to privacy. Patients enjoyed being involved in their plan of care and information.

Box 1.21 An example of a crossover trial involving pregnant women in Canada.

A crossover trial compared the tolerability and compliance rates of 138 pregnant women attending outpatient clinics in Ontario and Quebec who received two types of multivitamin supplements (Ahn et al., 2006). One supplement (PregVit®) contained a low dose of iron (35 mg) the other one (Materna®) contained a higher dose of iron (60 mg). Women were recruited at their first contact visit, asked to complete a standard questionnaire and randomised to receive either (PregVit®) or (Materna®) to be taken for 1 month. Women were asked to keep a diary of any adverse event (e.g. constipation, nausea and headache).One month later the supplement was changed over and given for 1 month. The results reported a significantly higher incidence of constipation as well as average duration of constipation when taking Materna®, the supplement containing a higher dose of iron when compared with PregVit®, the supplement containing a lower dose of iron.

However, this kind of trial cannot be used for treatments/interventions that have a permanent effect, and sometimes there has to be a time period between receiving the treatment/intervention. See Box 1.21.

Randomised controlled trials

Randomised controlled trials (RCTs) use an experimental design; a researcher investigates the effectiveness of two or more interventions/treatments in a number of individuals who have been randomly allocated to a control or experimental or standard regimen group. RCTs are considered to be a comparative study but the study must involve participants being allocated at

Box 1.22 An example of a randomised controlled trial.

Steen and Marchant (2007) carried out a RCT in a large maternity unit in the north of England. The aim of this RCT was to evaluate the effectiveness of two localised cooling treatments (ice pack and cooling gel pad) compared with a no localised treatment group at relieving perineal pain. Four hundred and fifty women who had either undergone a normal or instrumental delivery that required suturing of an episiotomy or second-degree tear were randomly assigned to one of the three treatment groups. The response rate was 316 out of 450 (71%). Perineal pain was most severe when sitting compared to lying down or walking and there was a significant difference between the three groups in estimates of overall pain when sitting on day four (Kruskal-Wallis test, $df = 2$ $p = 0.01$). Estimates of overall pain were lower in the gel pad group, and the difference between the three groups was significant at day five and day ten (Kruskal-Wallis test, $df = 2$ $p = 0.02$, $p = 0.01$). On days two, three and five, significance was measured when making a binary comparison of reported 'moderate' or 'severe' pain with 'none' or 'mild' (chi-square test, $p = 0.04$, $p = 0.04$, $p = 0.02$). Using a summary pain measurement, mothers experienced fewer painful days in the gel pad group but this did not reach statistical significance (Kruskal-Wallis test, $df = 2$ $p = 0.26$). The use of analgesia was reported to be similar in all three groups. Maternal satisfaction with their overall care was rated more highly in the gel pad group when compared to the two other groups (Kruskal-Wallis test, $df = 2$ $p > 0.001$). The conclusions were that cooling treatments can alleviate pain when compared to no localised treatment. Women appeared to find the cooling gel pad to be a more acceptable treatment.

random to an intervention/treatment group. RCTs measure and compare different outcomes when participants receive an intervention/treatment or not. An independent variable is manipulated to look for an effect on the dependent variable(s). RCTs are considered to be the most appropriate research method to investigate the effectiveness of a treatment or intervention and are the standard method of answering questions about the effectiveness of different treatments/interventions.

A randomised controlled study is one in which:

- There are two or more treatment/intervention groups (experimental) and a control group.
- The groups are 'like for like', i.e. they are similar in everything except the treatment/intervention they receive.
- The treatment/intervention group(s) receives the treatment/intervention under investigation, and the control group receives a no treatment, a standard regimen or placebo.
- Participants are randomly assigned to all groups.

See Box 1.22.

Box 1.23 An example of a cluster randomised controlled trial.

Moore *et al.* (2002) evaluated the effectiveness of a self-help approach to smoking in pregnancy. A cluster RCT with community midwife as the unit of randomisation was undertaken in three NHS hospital trusts in England; 1527 women who smoked at the beginning of pregnancy were recruited. A series of self-help booklets was given to the women by a midwife at the earliest opportunity in antenatal care and also a booklet for partners, family members and friends. Further booklets were mailed directly to the women. The primary outcome was smoking cessation validated by cotinine measurement at the end of the second trimester of pregnancy. Smoking cessation rates were low: the cotinine validated rates were 18.8% (113/600) in the intervention group and 20.7% (144/695) in the normal group (difference 1.9%, 95% confidence intervals −3.5% to 7.3%). Pregnant women and midwives approved of the intervention, but the way in which it was delivered varied considerably. The self-help intervention was acceptable but ineffective when implemented during routine antenatal care.

Assigning participants at random reduces the risk of bias and increases the probability that any differences between the groups can be attributed to the treatment/intervention. Having a control group allows us to compare the treatment/intervention with alternative choices. However, sometimes when undertaking research, RCTs cannot be carried out for ethical reasons, i.e. if there is risk of harm. See: Chapter 5, Ethics & Research Governance. An example of this would be randomising low-risk women to have a Caesarean section or vaginal delivery when there is no medical or obstetric indication for operative intervention.

Cluster trials
These randomise interventions/treatments to groups of participants rather than to individual participants. So the unit of measurement is the cluster and not the individual. Usually there is a larger sample size and the analysis is more complex. Ideally, cluster trials are suited to test interventions such as a community-based health programme. See Box 1.23.

The importance of evidence-based practice

Midwives have a professional responsibility to keep themselves up to date with the best available evidence. In the past, midwifery care has been based on traditional and cultural practices. Research was not included in the midwifery curriculum until the 1980s. Midwives then began to develop skills that enabled them to read, apply, understand and undertake research activities. It is now accepted that midwifery care can no longer be based on ritual and traditional practices and it must be supported by research evidence. An ethnographic study, however, that explored whether midwives are using research evidence to support clinical practice reported that the issues that impact on the integration of evidence into practice are complex and there are no straightforward answers (Richens, 2002).

The reality is that some traditional practices that have been handed down appear to have some value and some do not and it is about getting the balance right. An example of a practice that has been demonstrated to be harmful is the advice that was initially written by Dr Spock (an American paediatrician) in the book *Baby and Child Care* published in 1956. He advised that babies should be placed on their fronts when sleeping as there was a risk of aspiration of vomit and choking when babies are placed on their backs. In the 1970s it was common practice for premature babies to be placed in the prone position as it improved respiratory function in babies with respiratory distress and reduced vomiting in babies with gastro-oesophageal reflux. This influenced baby care practices on full-term healthy infants and babies were placed on their fronts in the postnatal wards. There was an increase in sudden infant death syndrome (SIDS) in the 1970s and 1980s; by reversing the advice, the 'back to sleep' initiative led to a dramatic decline in SIDS in the 1990s (Evans *et al.*, 2006). However, placing infants on their fronts, 'tummy time', is recommended when a baby is awake to offset motor skill delays associated with the 'back to sleep' position and plagiocephaly (flat head) (Majnemer & Barr, 2005).

These practices need to be evaluated and audit and research play an important part in assessing the benefits or not of the practices. Nevertheless, a multitude of professional and organisational constraints that prevent evidence-based practice (EBP) from being implemented has been acknowledged (Parahoo, 2009); that said the importance of EBP has increased and it is happening.

> An important aspect of evidence-based practice is the need to develop standardised measurable outcomes that allow the clinical practitioner to record the nature and severity of a given condition and then the effect of any care provided.
> Steen & Cooper, 1998, p. 6

A thorough, well designed systematic review and meta-analysis provides knowledge of the effectiveness of specific interventions/treatments but has limitations. Both quantitative and qualitative evidence need to be considered when implementing EBP. Other types of study designs are also needed to explore what is acceptable and structured reviews and meta-syntheses of qualitative evidence provide valuable information.

It has been recommended that students develop within a culture that encourages them to challenge clinical practice that is not supported by EBP (Royal College of Midwives (RCM), 2003; NMC, 2004b). However, there is evidence that what is taught during midwifery education and training does not always correspond to what is happening in midwifery practice. Armstrong (2010) has reported that midwifery students have a preference towards EBP but challenging their midwifery mentors, if they were not practising EBP, would be difficult to undertake for fear of jeopardising their clinical assessments and career prospects. Interestingly, a qualitative study undertaken by Stapleton *et al.* (2002), who used non-participant observation and semi-structured interviews to explore the use of evidence-based leaflets on informed choice in maternity services, found that many midwives initially expressed positive views about the principles underpinning the leaflets. However, the leaflets were rarely used to maximum effect within practice settings. Some women expressed dissatisfaction when written information was used as an alternative to discussion. It was concluded that the way in which the leaflets were disseminated affected promotion of informed choice in maternity care.

Evidence-based guidelines

Evidence-based guidelines are systematically developed to provide guidance and recommendations to assist health professionals and service users to make decisions about the most effective healthcare to treat or prevent specific clinical conditions. Clinical guidelines provide recommendations for effective practice in the management and care of the health and well-being of the population. Throughout the world there are variations in health and maternal care. There are clinical guidelines available, but these are often based on a consensus of expert opinion, traditional practices or a non-systematic review of the published literature. The importance of evidence-based guidelines has increased over the last decade; they are less susceptible to bias in their conclusions and recommendations. National guidelines funded by various departments of health and professional bodies are developing a resource of evidence-based reviews and reports. For example, the National Institute for Health & Clinical Excellence (NICE) guidelines have been used to develop policies and standards for midwifery practice in England and Wales.

The National Institute for Health and Clinical Excellence (NICE)

NICE was set up in early 1999 as a Special Health Authority and is an independent organisation in England and Wales responsible for providing national guidance on the promotion of good health and the prevention and treatment of ill health. See: http://www.nice.org.uk/. Northern Ireland also now utilises NICE guidelines to help make clinical decisions and the Guidelines and Audit Implementation Network (GAIN) has an important safety and quality improvement role in Health & Social Care Services. See http://www.gain-ni.org/.

NICE produces guidance in three areas of health:

- Public health – guidance on the promotion of good health and the prevention of ill health for those working in the NHS, local authorities and the wider public and voluntary sector.

- Health technologies – guidance on the use of new and existing medicines, treatments and procedures within the NHS.
- Clinical practice – guidance on the appropriate treatment and care of people with specific diseases and conditions within the NHS.

NICE guidance is developed using the expertise of the NHS and the wider healthcare community including service users (patients and carers), healthcare professionals, NHS staff, industry and the academic world. NICE categorises its guidance by health subject and date published.

NICE guidance aims are:

- To promote good health and prevent ill health.
- To produce guidance documents where a range of representatives have been involved and consulted, those being health and social care professionals, patients and the general public.
- To provide guidance based on the best evidence drawn from systematic reviews.
- To be transparent in the guidance development and use quality assessment tools to promote reliability and consistency.
- To weigh up the cost and benefits of treatments and care.
- To make recommendations based on the evidence.

Over a decade on and NICE is now internationally recognised for its excellence and the NICE model is being utilised in Europe (Busse & Worz, 2003). NICE International contributes to better health around the world through the more effective and equitable use of resources. It does this by providing advice on the use of evidence and social values in making clinical and policy decisions. In addition on-going evaluation and review of the implementation of NICE guidance documents is carried out to audit its effects on clinical practice by the Evaluation & Review of NICE Implementation Evidence (ERNIE). See http://www.nice.org.uk/usingguidance/evaluationandreviewofnice implementationevidenceernie/. Box 1.24 gives an example of NICE clinical guidelines.

Box 1.24 An example of NICE clinical guidelines – CG62 Issued March 2008.

Antenatal care: routine care for the healthy pregnant woman

The advice in the NICE guideline covers the routine care that all healthy women can expect to receive during their pregnancy.

It does not specifically look at women who are pregnant with more than one baby, women with certain medical conditions or women who develop a health problem during their pregnancy.

See http://www.guidance.nice.org.uk/CG62.

The Scottish Intercollegiate Guidelines Network (SIGN)

In Scotland, the Scottish Intercollegiate Guidelines Network (SIGN) was formed in 1993. SIGN develops evidence-based clinical practice guidelines for the NHS in Scotland. SIGN guidelines are developed from evidence gathered by systematic reviews and are designed to help bridge the theory–practice gap. The implementation of new knowledge into practice is the main objective of SIGN as this will reduce variations in practice and improve patient outcomes.

SIGN guidelines are developed by multidisciplinary working groups with professional and public representatives. Each guideline is based on the critical appraisal of the most up-to-date evidence. Evidence is identified, selected and evaluated according to a defined methodology. The guideline recommendations are graded according to the strength of the evidence. The ABCD grading score was developed from the original US Agency for Health Care Policy and Research approach to grading in its guidelines. (Evolved to become the Agency of Healthcare Research and Quality, AHRQ). SIGN guidelines, therefore, are based on a systematic review of the evidence, undertaken by guideline development groups which are supported by an executive.

SIGN guidelines are developed based on three core principles:

- Development is carried out by multidisciplinary, nationally representative groups.
- A systematic review is conducted to identify and critically appraise the evidence.
- Recommendations are explicitly linked to the supporting evidence.

For further information see http://www.sign.ac.uk/about/index.html.

Since 1 January 2005 SIGN has been part of NHS Quality Improvement Scotland (NHS QIS). NHS QIS is a special health board that advises, supports and assesses Scottish NHS boards to help improve the quality of healthcare which focuses broadly on safety, quality and health issues. There is a specific guidance on health improvement for maternal and child health and in March 2009, NHS QIS published the normal maternity care pathway which is based on the philosophy that pregnancy and childbirth are normal processes and unnecessary intervention should be avoided. The pathway supports the need to provide expectant mothers and their families with the most up-to-date evidence-based information. It recommends that a midwife should be the lead professional for healthy women with uncomplicated pregnancies. For further information see http://www.nhsqis.org/nhsqis/5205.141.1220.html.

Institute for Quality Assurance (IQA) Health and Social Care

IQA Health and Social Care has been established to bring together health professions and organisations that have an interest in continuously improving the quality of health and social care in the United Kingdom. The overall aim is to promote measurable and continuous improvement in the quality of health and social care for the benefit of the general public. It has strong links with NICE and the National Patient Safety Agency (NPSA).

The National Patient Safety Agency (NPSA)
In the UK, the NPSA leads and contributes to improved, safe patient care by informing, supporting and influencing the health sector. It commissions and monitors the Confidential Enquiry into Maternal and Child Health (CEMACH) which has now become Confidential Enquiry into Maternal and Child Enquiries (CMACE). See http://www.npsa.nhs.uk/.

Confidential Enquiry into Maternal and Child Enquiries (CMACE)
The overall aim of the Confidential Enquiry into Maternal and Child Enquiries (CMACE) is to improve the health of mothers, babies and children by carrying out confidential enquiries and related work. It has an important role in disseminating the findings and making recommendations.

An example: results from a survey on NHS maternity provision for obese women and guidelines on the Management of Obesity in Pregnancy (CMACE-RCOG, 2010).

See http://www.cmace.org.uk/.

The Agency of Healthcare Research and Quality (AHRQ)
AHRQ is funded by the US Department of Health and Human Services to support health services' research initiatives that aim to improve the quality of healthcare in America. AHRQ's mission is *'to improve the quality, safety, efficiency, effectiveness, and cost-effectiveness of health care for all Americans.'* For further information see http://www.ahrq.gov/.

The US Preventive Services Task Force (USPSTF) is sponsored by the AHRQ to conduct thorough independent reviews of the scientific evidence for the effectiveness of a wide range of clinical preventive services and interventions. Twelve Evidence-based Practice Centers (EPCs) have been established to work collaboratively with the AHRQ and USPSTF to develop evidence reports and technology assessments. Five-year contracts are awarded to institutions in the United States and Canada to serve as EPCs.

There is a specific Women's Health section and a Maternal Health and Pregnancy category (under clinical topics); an example report is The Use of Episiotomy in Obstetrical Care: A Systematic Review. This report provides the best available evidence on episiotomy use and concludes there are no health benefits from episiotomy. The full report can be downloaded as a PDF file from http://www.ahrq.gov/clinic/tp/epistp.htm#Report.

There is also a 'Consumer Materials' section which provides the evidence in lay person language, What you need to know about episiotomy...

Research shows that routine use of episiotomies (surgical cuts in the area between the vagina and anus) does not keep the mother's skin from tearing during birth.

It does not speed up a normal birth. It does not help avoid the bladder control problems women sometimes get after having a baby.

The consumer report can be downloaded from http://www.ahrq.gov/consumer/episiotomy.htm.

Evidence-Based Maternity Care: What It Is and What It Can Achieve

A very detailed report by Sakala and Corry and co-published by Childbirth Connection, the Reforming States Group, and the Milbank Memorial Fund (2008) entitled *Evidence-Based Maternity Care: What It Is and What It Can Achieve* gives in-depth information about current maternity care in the US healthcare system. The report summarises results of systematic reviews that could be used to improve maternity care and identifies barriers to the use of evidence-based maternity care. It offers policy recommendations and other strategies that could lead to wider implementation of evidenced-based maternity care in the US.

For further information visit http://www.milbank.org/reports/0809 MaternityCare/0809MaternityCare.html#executive.

National Antenatal Guidelines – Australia

The Australian government's Department of Health and Ageing works in collaboration with the National Health and Medical Research Council (NHMRC) to support health research in Australia. Clinical guidelines and health information leaflets based on the best available evidence are produced.

For Maternal and Infant Health see http://www.health.gov.au/internet/main/publishing.nsf/Content/phd-maternal-index.

Presently, National Evidence-Based Antenatal Care Guidelines are being developed. A collaboration of state and territory governments and the NHMRC with funding from the Australian Health Ministers' Advisory Council is supporting this work. The Antenatal Guidelines will be based upon the best available evidence to assist in the promotion of national standardisation of antenatal care and will include flexibility to meet individual needs to improve maternal and infant health outcomes. See http://www.health.gov.au/internet/main/publishing.nsf/Content/phd-antenatal-care-index.

Irish Society for Quality and Safety in Healthcare (ISQSH)

The ISQSH is a not-for-profit, charitable, non-governmental organisation whose overall aim is to improve the quality and safety of healthcare; it has set objectives to support the development of health professionals through professional education, training and research. In addition, it aims to provide a network for those working in or interested in healthcare quality. The society is governed by a multidisciplinary elected council and has strong collaborative links with a number of national and international partners including the

European and International Societies for Quality in Healthcare and the European Pathways Association. See http://www.isqsh.ie/.

European Society for Quality in Health Care (ESQH)
ESQH is a not-for-profit organisation dedicated to the improvement of quality in healthcare in Europe. Twenty national societies for quality in healthcare are members of this society, these include: Croatia, Czech Republic, Denmark, Finland, France, Germany, Greece, Ireland, Italy Lithuania, Luxembourg, The Netherlands, Norway, Poland, Portugal, Spain, Sweden, Turkey, United Kingdom and Egypt. See http://www.esqh.net/newsfolder_view? portal_status_title=ESQH+NEWS.

Summary

This first chapter has covered the general principles of research and given an insight into the types of knowledge, the research process, the difference between audit and research, the importance of the research question, the approaches that can be undertaken, the differences between these and the importance of applying evidence to midwifery care. Midwifery research has developed over the last few decades. The midwifery examples included in this chapter are only the tip of the iceberg and there is an ever increasing number of midwives and students developing research skills to undertake research activities. These examples demonstrate how both qualitative and quantitative research have been used to gather evidence to enhance midwifery care and practice. The different research methods that can be used to answer a specific research question have been introduced and the next chapters in this book will build upon this introduction to research.

In summary, this introductory chapter has set the scene; midwives and students should now be able to recognise different types of knowledge, know the difference between audit and research, be able to distinguish between qualitative and quantitative research approaches, will have gained knowledge and an understanding of different research methods and have an understanding of the importance of evidence-based practice. Service user involvement is considered good practice in all stages of research and this chapter highlights the importance of listening to women and their families; their ideas and views give an insight into what needs to be researched and how to conduct the research. Working in partnership with women and their families makes a difference to research outcomes and ultimately midwifery care and practice. It is now accepted that midwifery care can no longer be based on ritual and traditional practices and it must be supported by research evidence. Midwives have a professional responsibility to keep themselves up to date with the best available evidence. The next chapter gives an insight into how to perform this task.

CHAPTER 2

2 # Finding the evidence

Introduction to finding evidence

This chapter will focus on developing knowledge and understanding about how to find the evidence. Literature searching and identifying different sources of evidence will be explored, and the need to develop research skills and strategies to enable midwives and students to undertake a structured and systematic approach to finding the evidence will be discussed. Recent examples to demonstrate how these research activities have been used and how the evidence has impacted on clinical practice will be discussed further. This will highlight the effects of research evidence upon clinical practice.

Midwives and students will be encouraged to undertake a literature search and then use a search strategy to structure a review on a midwifery topic of their choice. After undertaking this task, midwives and students may even be inspired to undertake further research on their chosen topic and build upon this when studying and writing their research dissertation or thesis.

Aim
The aim of this chapter is to enable readers to gain knowledge and an understanding on how to find evidence by undertaking a literature search and identifying different sources of evidence. This will also involve developing research skills and strategies to assist student midwives to use a structured and systematic approach to their literature searching.

Learning outcomes

By the end of the chapter midwives and students:

- will have gained knowledge and skills of literature searching;
- will be able to recognise different sources of evidence;
- will have been guided to review data resources that are available;
- will be able to undertake a literature search on a topic of their choice;
- will have developed research skills to use a search strategy;
- will be able to undertake a structured and systematic approach to finding the evidence.

The Handbook of Midwifery Research, First Edition. Mary Steen and Taniya Roberts.
© 2011 Mary Steen and Taniya Roberts. Published 2011 by Blackwell Publishing Ltd.

Literature searching

Midwives and students have a responsibility to provide the best care possible and this has to be based on the most up-to-date evidence (NMC, 2008). For this, midwives and students will have to read a lot of information and know where and how to find the information. Most information is in some type of written or media format that can be easily accessed from a number of resources. Midwives and students will need to learn how to undertake a literature search, firstly to keep themselves up to date with the latest research evidence to inform their practice and, secondly, to study in depth an area of interest they wish to further explore and investigate.

What is a literature search?

A literature search is an in-depth search for information using several resources and tools to provide knowledge and an understanding of a specific topic of interest. The retrieved information will give an insight into what and how research has been undertaken, best available evidence, ongoing debates and disagreements and what are the gaps and areas for further research.

There are numerous journals, guidelines, policies and reviews that publish relevant and up-to-date information but it is often difficult for midwives and students to access the vast amount of information with all the other personal and professional commitments they have to meet. These difficulties contribute to the theory–practice gap. Fortunately, there are some journals and resources that summarise the latest events, news and relevant reports, but to review a subject in-depth it will take a lot of time, motivation and skills to search all the relevant information. The use of computers, access to electronic databases, journals and the internet in the clinical areas, in academic institutions and the availability of remote access when undertaking undergraduate and postgraduate studies can help you balance work, study and your personal life.

Literature review

A literature review is an in-depth review of all sources of information available on a topic of interest that has then been critically analysed, giving a summary of all key landmark findings and most up-to-date evidence, the gaps and unresolved issues are identified, and the evidence is evaluated and presented in a written report prior to undertaking a research study or implementing evidence-based guidelines, policies and revising pathways of care.

Hart (2005, p. 13) defines a literature review in similar terms:

> The selection of available documents (both published and unpublished) on the topic, which contain information, ideas, data and evidence written from a particular standpoint to fulfil certain aims or express certain views on the nature of the topic and how it is to be investigated, and the effective evaluation of these documents in relation to the research being proposed.

However, it has to be acknowledged that a reviewer needs to be objective in their views, findings and evaluation of the information as far as possible. To do this it is important to recognise a particular standpoint you may have, your predetermined thoughts and judgements, and your cultural and social background, beliefs and attitudes concerning the area of interest. Being aware of how these factors can influence the review and acknowledging them as limitations will enable a reviewer to demonstrate that they have considered their personal biases and have the ability to show what is commonly referred to as **reflexivity** in research.

Undertaking a literature review can be a time-consuming and challenging task. A lack of knowledge and understanding of how to use a library's facilities and information and communication technologies (ICTs) at the commencement of a research study is a common phenomenon. Specific knowledge and an appreciation of how to search and understand library indexes, catalogues, e-learning resources, databases and e-journals needs to be mastered. For example, you will need to become familiar with MeSH® terms. MeSH stands for Medical Subject Headings and is the US National Library of Medicine's (NLM) controlled vocabulary thesaurus. The MeSH thesaurus is used by NLM for indexing articles from 5200 of the world's leading biomedical journals for the MEDLINE/PubMED® database. MeSH uses word and term descriptors that are arranged in an alphabetical and hierarchical structure that permits searching at various levels of specificity. Broad and specific terms can be used and an awareness of these will help you search MEDLINE/PubMED®. A useful MeSH factsheet is freely available to download from: http:// www.nlm.nih.gov/pubs/factsheets/mesh.html.

You will also need to know how a database record is structured and become familiar with specific abbreviations that are used, which can be a task in itself. All on-line databases use some form of structured format but differ in their styles. Box 2.1 an example of an on-line structured record of a journal article.

Whilst undertaking the search many midwives and students have a tendency to become easily distracted and end up looking at information that is not directly relevant to their subject of interest, but nevertheless, they find this information interesting in itself and relevant to midwifery practice. Often valuable time is wasted and there is a lesson to be learned here. When undertaking a literature review set strict guidelines at the outset and if you find you are digressing, quickly recognise this, reflect and refocus on what you are specifically reviewing, stay within certain boundaries, use time lines and tick off tasks as you complete them (Table 2.1). It is essential that you learn some search management skills as part of the process and develop your own useful aids. Checklists, mind maps and time charts will help you to progress logically and in a structured productive way. Basically, the core skills you will need to develop include time management, computer skills, how to do on-line searches, how to organise and manage the data and how to critically analyse and write your review (Hart, 2005).

Box 2.1 An example of an on-line structured record of a journal article in Maternity & Infant Care Database.

Record 1 of 8 in Maternity & Infant Care October 2007

AU: Moyle-M; Moore-EJ; Varigos-G
TI: Characteristic adverse skin reactions to antiseptic bath oils
SO: Medical Journal of Australia vol 186 no 12 pp 652–653
JN: Medical-Journal-of-Australia
PY: 2007
DE: Anti-infective-agents-local; Infant-; Oils-; Skin-care
ST: Skin-Care-of-Newborn
SC: PN83
IS: 0025-729X
DT: Journal-article
PT: Case-report
AI: Y
AB: Presents three case reports with accompanying photos of acute contact
   dermatitis after bathing in antiseptic bath oil. (6 references) (MB)
AN: 3455; 2007070549
UD: 20070717
VO: vol 186
NO: 12
FP: 652
LP: 653

Table 2.1 Checklist for literature reviewing.

Management of literature search	Tools and techniques
Seek advice and support	Attend relevant study sessions, days, workshops
Develop structured plan	Gain hands-on experience and practice of searching
Be systematic in your approach	databases
Make a list of tasks to do and tick (✓) them off when completed	Develop your own list of instructions on how to use ICTs
Keep a log of all your review activities and check progress at regular intervals (weekly/monthly)	Develop a system for organising and storing each source of information
Good recording keeping is paramount	Dichotomise articles to either relevant or not relevant
Document the search title, keywords, terms and phrases used	Categorise information, i.e. research study, editorial, review, commentary or discussion paper, audit report, policy or guideline documents etc.
Record time of search and time period specified	Citations and references (can be indexed manually or electronically)
Keep a printed copy of every electronic database searched and the numbers of articles found and retrieved	Find out what software packages are available to record citations and references, i.e. ProCite and Endnote
	Keep a research diary – to reflect on your learning

Know your topic of interest

Once an in-depth search of the literature has been undertaken and all relevant sources of information have been retrieved, the next task is to become familiar with the knowledge and gain an understanding of the available evidence and key issues. This task involves critically analysing the retrieved information and then writing up a report that includes introducing the subject, describing and discussing the evidence, highlighting any key landmark studies and recent studies, the debates and unresolved issues identified, and your own critical thoughts and evaluation of the collective evidence gathered. This task is necessary to complete the literature review and is discussed in greater detail in the Chapter 3, Making Sense of the Evidence.

Sources of evidence

There are several resources available to identify background information and the most up-to-date evidence but you may feel overwhelmed in the first instance just by the amount of information there is out there; don't panic! This is a normal reaction and you will ask yourself where do I start? You need to develop a **plan of work** that covers your **learning needs** and **area of interest**. Who can help you? Your tutors, a supervisor if you are undertaking a dissertation or thesis and, very importantly, a librarian who specialises in health studies may all be of assistance. These people can help guide you as to where to look for the information, and can suggest the most suitable databases, websites, latest published maternity policies etc., and then how to sort the information retrieved, decide what is relevant, of good quality and what to disregard. You will develop skills in literature searching and how to use search tools as you undertake the search.

The Cochrane Library

The Cochrane Library is a collection of databases that contain high-quality, independent evidence to inform healthcare decision-making. Health professionals and the general public can freely access the Cochrane Library via the internet.

The Cochrane Collaboration Trials Register and Systematic Reviews are good sources of information and represent the highest level of evidence on which to base clinical treatment/intervention decisions. The Cochrane Library also provides other sources of reliable information to help promote evidence-based practice. See the Cochrane Library on-line at http://www.cochrane.org/reviews/clibintro.htm.

The Cochrane Collaboration

The Cochrane Collaboration, founded in 1992, is an international not-for-profit organisation, which provides the latest information on the effects of healthcare and treatments. The Collaboration's vision is that:

Healthcare decision-making around the world will be informed by high-quality and timely research evidence. The collaboration will play a pivotal role in the production and dissemination of this evidence across all areas of health care.

Cochrane Pregnancy and Childbirth Group

The Cochrane Collaboration has set up numerous review groups and assesses most areas of healthcare. The first review group was in fact the Cochrane Pregnancy and Childbirth Group which was originally based in Oxford and was developed from the pioneering work on systematic reviews by Sir Iain Chalmers and colleagues. In 1995, the review group moved to Liverpool and systematic reviews were published and available electronically in the Cochrane Database of Systematic Reviews, which is now published in the Cochrane Library. Recently, a sub-review group has been set up in Australia.

In addition, reviews of relevance to developing countries have also now been published electronically in the Reproductive Health Library and the World Health Organization supports the dissemination of the evidence to developing countries. See the following website link for detailed information: http://www.mrw.interscience.wiley.com/cochrane/clabout/articles/PREG/frame.html.

Midwives Information & Resource Service (MIDIRS) Reference Database (formerly Maternity and Infant Care)

This specifically focused midwifery/maternity and infant care database was first developed in 1988 and has access to around 550 international English language health journals which are frequently scanned to update the evidence on this database. Evidence has been collected from 1973 to present and covers journal articles, book chapters, reports, any news, audiovisual resources, conference events and other 'grey literature' relating to the midwifery profession and maternity and infant care.

This maternity reference database is a very useful database to use as a starting point and then you can continue to search other specific health-related electronic databases such as CINAHL, MEDLINE, EMBASE, Intute etc. You may need a password or an Athens account to access these so check this with your library and what e-learning resources are available for you to use.

Other databases

Useful bibliographic databases include:

- **CINAHL** – major bibliographic database for nursing and allied health;
- **MEDLINE** – major bibliographic database for biomedical sciences (Pubmed searches MEDLINE and other life science journals for biomedical articles back to the 1950s);
- **EMBASE** – major bibliographic database for biomedical sciences;
- **Intute** – major bibliographic database for biomedical sciences.

Depending on your topic and what information you want to include in your review you may need to search specific databases such as:

- **AMED** – Allied and Complementary Medicine Database;
- **BNI** – the British Nursing Index;
- **PsychINFO** – major bibliographic database for psychology;
- **NHS Evidence** is developing and if you have access to this database you will be able to combine some of the database searches.

In the UK, the recently developed NHS Evidence resource, collaboratively produced by NICE (The National Institute for Health and Clinical Excellence) and NLH (The National Library for Health) is an attempt to simplify finding research evidence to support best clinical practice. It aims to provide easy internet access to the best available evidence for health professionals using only one search engine and has a very useful function of being able to combine several database searches into one (Holly, 2009; NHS, 2009). For further information see http://www.evidence.nhs.uk/

In addition, another possible useful resource available via NHS Evidence is the **Map of Medicine** which has an Obstetric and Gynaecology section. For example, if you want to find information about a clinical pathway for Caesarean section, see the following weblink: http://nhsevidence.mapofmedicine.com/evidence/map/caesarean_section1.html.

The **James Lind Library** is also an excellent resource. It has been developed to increase public and professional general knowledge about how 'fair' tests can help us to distinguish helpful from harmful effects of treatments. If you want to review historical research then this website is very useful and is available in several different languages (English, Arabic, Chinese, French, Portuguese, Russian and Spanish). See weblink http://www.jameslindlibrary.org/library.html.

Within the area of interest you have chosen, you will need to decide what exactly the question is you want to answer. You may want to update a care pathway; to do this you need to have a general knowledge base and understanding of the latest research findings, the interpretations, expert opinions, recommendations, differences in approaches to care, and which national guidelines and policies are currently in existence and which can inform clinical practice. Alternatively, you may be wanting to test out a theory or a new treatment/intervention and need to undertake a specifically focused search of the literature; in this case you need to use a search strategy.

Other helpful services
- **The Joanna Briggs Institute** – this is an international organisation specialising in evidence-based resources for healthcare professionals: http://www.joannabriggs.edu.au/.
- **Intermid.co.uk** – this service provides articles from British Journal of Midwifery and from African Journal of Midwifery and Women's Health: http://www.intermid.co.uk/.
- **Intute: Nursing Midwifery & Allied Health** – this service provides help to find websites for studying and research: http://www.intute.ac.uk/nmah/.

- **ScienceDirect** – this service provides articles from several nursing, midwifery, health and medical journals: http://www.sciencedirect.com/.
- **RCM Midwifery website** – this service provides articles from Midwives magazine, on-line papers, Evidence-Based Midwifery journal and has a Student e-zine resource: http://www.rcm.org.uk/.
- **Midwifery mkn** – the Midwifery Managed Knowledge Network (MKN) is a service that enables midwives to access and share evidence-based information to support their care of new and expectant mothers: http://www.midwiferymkn.scot.nhs.uk/home.aspx.
- **Proquest** – this is an international datebase of graduate dissertations and theses: http://www.proquest.com/en-US/catalogs/databases/detail/pqdt.shtml.
- **Scopus** – this is an international database of literature citations and web resources: http://info.scopus.com/.

Using a search strategy

A search strategy is a well thought out approach and plan about to how to search for relevant information. It is essential to develop a search strategy that allows you to narrow down your search to something that is manageable.

You will have to decide what **time period** you will need to cover, the **type of information** you want to include and identify and make a list of the **keywords**, **terms** and **phrases** you want to use before searching electronic databases such as Medline and CINAHL. You will need to check the relevant periodical indexes and abstracts and make a note of the last index (issue) published and the time of your search.

Once you have a list of the keywords, terms and phrases, you can then link them by what are referred to as 'Boolean' words: AND, OR, NOT. 'AND' will help to narrow the search, in contrast 'OR' will broaden the search and 'NOT' will eliminate a word, term or phrase and narrow the search.

If you are using **permutations** (arrangement of words) in a database search, you must remember to put these in brackets and phrases need to be in quotation marks. See Box 2.2.

In addition, you need to take into consideration the different spellings used in UK and the US. Some midwifery and medical words are spelt differently, such as Caesarean and you will need to include different spellings, for example, Cesarean or Cesarian. Consider different permutations (arrangements) relating to words; for example, for breech, you would need to include frank or complete or extended or flexed.

You may find what is referred to as **truncating** (trim or abbreviate) helpful. This means using the base of a word and adding an asterisk (*) to find any words that begin with that base, for example midwif* = midwife, midwives, midwifery. You may also find **wildcards** helpful. These are symbols you can use to replace one or more characters in a word to cover plurals, for example father? = father, fathers.

Box 2.2 An example of a search strategy.

At present there is an ongoing debate regarding the evidence to support the most safe and effective mode of delivery for breech presentation. This debate instigated one of the authors and a colleague to carry out a search of the published literature and the implications this has had on clinical practice over the last 50 years (Steen & Kingdon, 2008a). The search strategy was specifically designed to identify research studies and commentary papers relating to the controversy surrounding whether breech presentations should be delivered vaginally or by planned Caesarean section.

Literature was identified by systematically searching the Cochrane Library (Issue 2008), CINAHL (1982 to 2008 week 5), EMBASE (1980 to 2008 week 5) and MEDLINE (1950 to 2008 week 5). Different permutations of 'breech' ('frank' or 'complete' or 'extended' or 'flexed') AND 'vaginal' OR 'Caesarean' ('Caesarean' or 'Cesarian' or 'Cesarean') AND 'term' AND 'singleton' in the title, keywords or abstracts were used.

Having a search strategy will help you to remain focused on your subject and within the limits of what you want to search.

Structured review

A structured review is a well organised review of the literature which involves the planning of a well thought out search strategy and has a specific focus and identifies what type of information within a specified timeframe is to be sought, critiqued and reported.

Examples of structured reviews
Breech birth: reviewing the evidence for external cephalic version and moxibustion (Steen & Kingdon, 2008b)

This structured review focused specifically on women's preferences for birth mode, experiences of breech presentation and the use of external cephalic version (ECV) and moxibustion, which may be used in the third trimester of pregnancy to turn a breech baby to a cephalic presentation.

The search strategy sought information from the Cochrane Library (Issue 1 2008), CINAHL (1982 to 2008 week 5), EMBASE (1980 to 2008 week 5) and MEDLINE (1950 to 2008 week 5) and AMED (1985 to February 2008). Different permutations of 'breech' ('frank' or 'complete' or 'extended' or 'flexed') AND alternative OR complementary therapies OR 'external cephalic version' OR 'ECV' OR 'moxibustion' AND 'before term' AND 'term' AND 'singleton' in the title, keywords or abstract were used.

The search strategy identified a total of 681 articles of which 283 abstracts were reviewed independently by the authors and 239 were excluded. A total of 44 potential papers were identified: four Cochrane reviews, eight systematic or structured reviews, ten reports on the findings of randomised controlled trials, 16 prospective studies, two retrospective studies and four commentaries. Following the authors' full reading of these potential papers a further 12 were excluded. A further four papers were identified through reference lists and hand searching, thus a total of 36 papers were reviewed. The studies identified varied in their quality and the best available evidence was provided by the Cochrane's reviews and systematic/structured reviews.

The authors reported that there is evidence that the majority of women would prefer a vaginal birth. There is substantial evidence that ECV can reduce the Caesarean section rate by turning breech presentation to cephalic. Further research is needed to confirm or refute the clinical effectiveness and women's views of moxibustion therapy.

The authors concluded that as rates of Caesarean section for breech presentation continue to rise it is important that midwives and women have up-to-date evidence-based information about the alternative to proceeding straight to planned Caesarean section when a breech presentation is identified.

A review of baby skin care (Steen & Macdonald, 2008) undertaken on behalf of the Royal College of Midwives, UK

This structured review, focused specifically on the skin and its functions, compared the skin of a full-term newborn baby to that of an adult skin and current evidence and opinions of experts to support best practice on baby skin care. This information was used to develop a list of good practice guidelines for midwives to use to help them inform and support parents.

The search strategy sought information from the Cochrane Central Register of Controlled Trials and Cochrane Database of Systematic Reviews and the National Research Register to identify any trials or systematic reviews investigating the use of baby skin care products, procedures or policies. A search of empirical articles using MEDLINE, CINAHL, EMBASE (January 1996 to November 2007) and keywords and terms ('baby', 'babies', 'infant'), AND 'skin' AND 'care', were used.

The search strategy initially, identified 550 CINAHL, 109 EMBASE and 293 MEDLINE articles; combining the keywords reduced the number of relevant articles to 22 CINAHL, 79 EMBASE and 33 MEDLINE. In addition a search of the Maternity and Infant Care database using the key words, infant and skin care produced a further 21 records.

The abstracts were reviewed by both authors to decide whether the article described a study or a systematic review on baby skin care products, procedures or polices relating to the full-term newborn to be included in this review.

Two randomised controlled trials were identified but on review of the full publication one of these was excluded as it was not published in the English language. One publication discussed the undertaking of two systematic reviews, one publication reported the findings from a postal survey and one publication discussed a large prospective study that investigated the effectiveness of clinical guidelines. The references given in these relevant articles were further examined. During a hand search the World Health Organization's (WHO) *Managing Newborn Problems* guidelines (WHO, 2003) and the recent National Institute of Health and Clinical Excellence (NICE) Guidelines on Postnatal Care (NICE, 2006) were identified. In addition, from the abstracts, 16 relevant articles were identified that discussed the skin and its functions, compared the skin of a full-term newborn baby to that of an adult skin or highlighted experts' opinions to support best practice on baby skin care. These were critically analysed, discussed and debated in the review and assisted in the development of guidelines.

The authors concluded that there is a lack of research studies investigating the use of baby skincare products, policies or procedures and there appears to be no consensus at present, as to whether to use water alone for the first 2–4 weeks of life or to use cleansers and moisturisers that are very mild and pH neutral.

The full text of the article is available on-line at http://www.rcm.org.uk/midwives/in-depth-papers/a-review-of-baby-skin-care/.

Systematic review

A systematic review involves reviewing quantitative studies, usually controlled trials that have investigated a specific treatment or intervention. The evidence is assessed to confirm or refute if a treatment or intervention is effective or not, or may even cause harm. Initially, all relevant trials are identified, and then critiqued. A quality assessment of the trials needs to be undertaken and, if they are deemed to be of good quality and biases have been addressed, the results from these trials can be combined and further statistical analysis may be undertaken which is known as *meta-analysis*. **Meta-analysis** produces an overall statistical result of the combined results collected from the individual trials that have been assessed as good quality (see Box 2.3). A systematic review is systematic in its approach and uses a predetermined and precise methodology to select the trials for inclusion and further analysis. A systematic review may not always include a meta-analysis of combined results due to the trials being dissimilar in their study design and the outcomes having been measured differently, i.e. different scales and time intervals.

When commencing a systematic review you have to develop a research protocol which outlines the question to be answered and a proposal detailing the methods.

A systematic review involves (NHMRC, 1999):

- question formulation;
- finding studies;
- appraisal and selection of studies;

Box 2.3 A Cochrane systematic review and meta-analysis (landmark research). Cochrane logo used with permission from The Cochrane Collaboration.

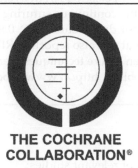

THE COCHRANE
COLLABORATION®

The Cochrane Collaboration logo demonstrates visually the results of a meta-analysis of data from seven clinical trials. These trials investigated the effectiveness of a steroid drug given to women who were expected to give birth prematurely. However, cumulative evidence from these trials was not known, as no systematic review of these trials was published until 1989 (Crowley, 1989). This Cochrane meta-analysis clearly shows that steroids reduce the risk of babies dying from the complications of immaturity. As no systematic reviews had been done, tens of thousands of premature babies suffered and died unnecessarily and resources were wasted on unnecessary research.

Basically, the seven horizontal lines represent the results of the trials and the diamond represents their combined results. The vertical line indicates the point around which the seven lines would come together if the treatments compared in the trials had similar effects. If the lines cross, it basically means that the trial found no clear statistically significant difference between the treatments. When a horizontal line crosses the vertical line (no difference), it suggests that the treatment might either increase or decrease infant deaths. The diagram shows that the horizontal lines tend to fall on the beneficial (left) side of the vertical 'no difference' line. The diamond represents the combined results of the trials of the meta-analysis. The position of the diamond clearly to the left of the vertical 'no difference' line indicates that the treatment is beneficial (Editorial commentary, 2007).

A Cochrane Collaboration systematic review undertaken by Kettle *et al.* (2007) assessed the effects of continuous versus interrupted absorbable sutures for repair of episiotomy and second-degree tears following childbirth. The reviewers searched the Cochrane's pregnancy and childbirth group's trials register for randomised controlled trials. Seven studies involving 3822 women from four countries were included in the review, and meta-analysis showed that continuous suture techniques compared with interrupted sutures for perineal closure are associated with less pain for up to 10 days postpartum (relative risk (RR) 0.70, 95% confidence interval (CI) 0.64–0.76). Subgroup analysis demonstrated that there is a

Continued

greater reduction in pain when continuous suturing techniques are used for all layers (RR 0.65, 95% CI 0.60– 0.71). An overall reduction in analgesia use was associated with the continuous suturing technique (RR 0.70, 95% CI 0.58–0.84) and also less dyspareunia (RR 0.83, 95% CI 0.70–0.98). A reduction in suture removal was also reported (RR 0.54, CI 95% 0.45– 0.65), but no differences between suture techniques were seen for re-suturing or long-term pain. See weblink http://www2.cochrane.org/reviews/en/ab000947.html.

- summary and synthesis of relevant studies;
- determining the applicability of results;
- reviewing and appraising economic literature.

Studies vary in quality, so it is helpful to use some form of systematic and standardised approach to how to appraise the studies to reduce study selection bias. A comprehensive and clear summary of the studies deemed to be of a high quality will assist midwives and students to review the evidence and this can support their practice.

In addition, an economic evaluation may be undertaken to provide evidence of costs and benefits of a service, treatment or intervention (NHMRC, 2000).

Summary

This chapter has focused on how to find the evidence. It has covered how to undertake a literature review, the sources of evidence available, how to use a search strategy and gives some useful examples. An insight into how to develop research skills and strategies to enable midwives and students to undertake structured and systematic searches to find the evidence has been discussed in an attempt to promote a better understanding of how to undertake a review. Examples have been included to demonstrate how evidence has been used and impacted on midwifery clinical practice.

The chapter has covered literature searching, some useful tools and resources available for midwives and students to use. It has included some useful guidance on how to undertake literature searching and this hopefully will help midwives and students to develop skills and clear strategies to manage the evidence identified and collected. The use of computers and the internet with remote access facilities and on-line access to databases and journals has assisted to make literature searching easier.

It is envisaged that midwives and students will now be able to confidently undertake a literature search using a wide variety of data resources on a topic of their choice. The literature review should include using a search strategy and a structured format to present the literature search findings. The information gathered will give an insight into what, where, when, why and how research has been undertaken. It will identify any ongoing controversies and debates and also where there are gaps and areas for further research.

Once midwives and students have successfully completed a literature search and identified the relevant studies and evidence to support their chosen topic of interest they will need to be able to critique and grade the quality of the research studies and evidence. The next chapter's focus will cover critiquing research studies and evidence.

3 Making sense of the evidence

Introduction to critiquing research evidence

This chapter will focus on how to critique research evidence and will highlight useful tools available. This information will assist midwives and students to undertake critiquing research evidence in a structured and systematic way. Critiquing both qualitative and quantitative research will be explored and discussed. Research evidence and how this is classified in levels of quality by using structured hierarchy of evidence tools will be included to assist student midwives to interpret the evidence. The differences between qualitative and quantitative methods and evidence will be further discussed and explored.

Aim

The aim of this chapter is to explore and develop research critiquing skills to assist midwives and students in implementing evidence-based practice.

Learning outcomes

By the end of this chapter midwives and students:

- will have gained knowledge and skills of critiquing research evidence;
- will be able to critique qualitative research;
- will be able to critique quantitative research;
- will be able to classify evidence;
- will be able to utilise this knowledge and skills to implement evidence-based practice.

Why critical appraisal is important

Critical appraisal is important because (NMC, 2008):

- midwives are involved in finding and evaluating evidence about the effectiveness of their practice and interventions;

The Handbook of Midwifery Research, First Edition. Mary Steen and Taniya Roberts.
© 2011 Mary Steen and Taniya Roberts. Published 2011 by Blackwell Publishing Ltd.

- in recent years, the importance of evidence-based practice (EBP) has been recognised;
- midwives have a professional responsibility to keep themselves up to date with the best available evidence;
- midwives can no longer base their role and responsibilities on rituals and traditional practices, they must be supported by evidence.

Research is used to support the decision-making processes of midwifery services (Hamer, 1999). Research involves a process of critically reflecting on past knowledge and traditional practices, then undertaking further investigative work which will promote the development of new understanding that can be used to inform clinical practice and improve standards of midwifery care (Steen, 2004).

Three questions to ask yourself are:

- Has the research been carried out correctly?
- Are the research methods and findings of the research relevant to your practice?
- Should you apply what was learned by the researcher to your practice?

Critically appraising a research study

Basically, a research study involves three stages:

- understanding the purpose of the study and considering if the way the research was designed appears to be consistent with purpose;
- studying how the research was actually carried out and deciding if it seems to have been done properly;
- seeing the findings of the research and judging if the conclusions reached are supported by the evidence.

Adapted from Critical Appraisal Skills Programme (CASP) (2006) and Crombie (2004).

Critiquing qualitative research

The word critiquing can summon up the image of someone appraising a research article for faults only. Critical appraisal however does in fact refer to a balanced scrutiny of a research paper, highlighting its strengths and weaknesses. A process can be followed and this usually takes the format of a critical appraisal framework (Rees, 2003), which aids the examination of the research article.

Today a newly qualified midwife will have been taught critical appraisal skills as part of his/her midwifery curriculum and will have become familiar with a variety of frameworks available. What must, however, be clearly understood is that there are different frameworks available dependent upon whether a qualitative or quantitative approach is adopted.

The structured process in Table 3.1 has been developed to help you critically appraise a qualitative study. The technique is to examine each section

Table 3.1 Critiquing a qualitative research paper.

The study	Questions
Publication	Do you think the journal that the study has been published in reaches its target audience?
	Is it midwifery specific?
	Is the study in date, i.e. from the completion of the study to publication, no longer than 3 years?
Title	Is it clear, succinct and understandable?
Abstract	Is it a concise overview of the study?
	Does it address the research question, outline the methodology, describe the sample, depict the findings and state any limitations?
	Does it capture the reader's attention and make you want to read the rest of the publication?
	The length of the abstract is determined by the journal in which it is published, usually 100–150 words; does it meet this requirement?
Author/s	Who are the authors?
	Are their qualifications, past publications or current posts detailed in the article and do they give them the credentials to conduct this research?
Funding	How has the study been funded?
	Could this be interpreted as biasing the study, depending on where it is from?
Introduction	Does it give a clear rationale of why the research study was conducted?
	Is the research question or aim clearly stated?
	Does it identify why the research question needed to be answered?
	Does it provide a contextual focus (background) for the research?
Literature review	Is it in date? (This usually refers to a 5-year window; however pivotal studies in the topic area are acceptable)
	Has the most recent research evidence been examined to provide a balanced argument to either support or challenge the proposed research?
	Has the review identified a gap in knowledge, i.e. that no research has been conducted on this topic in this way? This gives a very strong rationale for the study to be carried out
	Has the review identified dated research that could be duplicated?
	Has the review clearly identified the need for this study?
	Has any research been omitted from the literature review discussion? (When conducting a research critique, you should perform your own literature search to reach this conclusion)
	Does the review make sense?
Methodology	Does it state which research paradigm has been followed?
	Does it identify which research approach has been utilised – in this instance it should be the qualitative approach?
	If the above are not mentioned do you think the authors have made assumptions about their readers that they should know? Is it an assumption or omission on their part?
	Does it evidently describe the research methodology they are using, e.g. phenomenology?
	Are the description of and why the research methodology is utilised understandable to you?
	Have the authors clearly rationalised their use of it as opposed to others?

Table 3.1 *Continued*

The study	Questions
Sample	Is the type of sampling clearly stated? Does it match the research methodology that has been chosen? (e.g. phenomenology and purposive sampling) Is the sample size stated, do you consider this is an appropriate number? Is the sample size justified? Are inclusion/exclusion criteria explained and therefore do you understand why this sample was chosen? Is there an explanation of how the sample was recruited?
Method/data collection	Which method of data collection was utilised? Is it clearly explained? Does it match the research methodology? (Different methodologies utilise different data collection methods) Was the most appropriate method chosen? Is the concept of Saturation referred to? (i.e. when no new information is forthcoming data collection ceases) Is the notion of reflexivity expressed by the authors?
Data management	Are the procedures for managing the collected data described? Have computer software packages been used for this purpose?
Data analysis	Is the data analysis method clearly explained? Does it match the research methodology? (Different methodologies utilise different data analysis frameworks) Are the concepts of trustworthiness evident in this process? Has the researcher practised reflexivity? (referred to as putting aside personal biases)
Ethical considerations	Does it state that ethical approval has been gained? Does it state that informed consent was gained from the participants? Is participant confidentiality maintained? Does it explain how the collected data will be stored and destroyed after the completion of the study? Is the research process transparent, open to scrutiny? Have the researchers referred to an audit trail that could be followed by other researchers to establish the credibility of this research?
Findings	What are the findings? Do they address or answer the research question? Are the findings credible? How are the findings displayed, are there too little or too many quotes from the participants? Do the findings make sense?
Discussion	Does the discussion highlight the findings and link them to other studies in the same topic area? Does the discussion stress the significance of the study's findings and make recommendations for practice? Are any limitations referred to? Do you consider there were limitations to this study? Do you consider that the authors have over-stressed the significance of their study?
Conclusion	Does the conclusion neatly round up the research study, summing up the results of the study and the discussion?

of the research design and answer the questions posed. Once the questions have been answered you should then draw your own conclusion on the readability of the article and you should also consider whether the research study critiqued is a credible contribution to the body of midwifery research.

Meta-synthesis

Meta-synthesis is an in-depth analysis of published qualitative studies on a given subject and the method can generate new insights and understandings. Meta-synthesis attempts to integrate findings from a number of different but inter-related qualitative studies. The findings can then result in theory building, theory explanation and substantive descriptions of phenomena (Walsh & Downe, 2005; Barnett-Page & Thomas, 2009). Concerns, however, have been voiced about summarising qualitative research studies as there is a range of methodologies (Sandelowski *et al.*, 1997). Walsh and Downe (2006) suggest that concerns should be weighed against the consequences of not summarising qualitative research.

An increasing number of meta-synthesis papers are appearing in the midwifery literature (Clemmens, 2003; Kennedy *et al.*, 2003; Walsh & Downe, 2006; Downe *et al.*, 2007) and there appears to be a lack of consensus about some of the aspects of meta-synthesis. Walsh and Downe (2006) developed a framework to assess qualitative research after concluding that the ones that exist are *'excessively detailed'* and appraisal templates rather lengthy for most uses. The framework covers eight stages with essential criteria and specific prompts to guide a reviewer. The stages cover the aspects of:

- scope and purpose;
- design;
- sampling strategy;
- analysis;
- interpretation;
- reflexivity;
- ethical dimension;
- relevance and transferability.

This framework has helped one of the authors and two other midwifery researchers to develop a tool to undertake an assessment of qualitative papers relating to 'Involving Fathers in Maternity Care'. The three reviewers individually reviewed a full paper and then, collectively, through discussion came to an agreed grade and whether to include the study in a meta-synthesis, i.e. studies grade C+ or above were included. See Tables 3.2–3.5.

Meta-synthesis is an important technique for qualitative researchers and can deepen understanding of the contextual dimensions of midwifery care. It does have some similarities as well as differences to meta-analysis of quantitative studies.

Table 3.2 Initial screening (full text papers).

Code	Author/date	Reports fathers' views	Includes data on experiences of maternity care (up to 6 months P/N)	Includes qualitative data	IN?	Reviewer and date

COMMENTS:

Y = Yes, N = No, U = Unclear

Table 3.3 Characteristics of included studies and authors' findings.

Code	Author (year)	Aim(s)	Theoretical perspective	Study design	Sample selection method	Sample size and characteristics	Method of data collection	Method of data analysis	Reviewer date

KEY FINDINGS:

COMMENTS:

Y = Yes, N = No, U = Unclear, NA = Not appropriate

Critiquing quantitative research

Developing skills to undertake critical appraisal of research papers is important. Critical appraisal skills help a reviewer to appreciate the importance of good quality evidence. To assist with critically appraising quantitative research, checklists that provide some general and then more specific questions to ask when reviewing a published paper can be helpful. Checklists promote a structured approach to critiquing and a reviewer can systematically work through the questions to help them appraise the research in an orderly fashion. This approach gives a clear pathway and helps a reviewer to identify whether the research has been well designed and conducted and whether there are any limitations. This will assist the reviewer in making a decision as to whether the research provides evidence or not of a benefit to the study population.

Critical Appraisal Skills Programme (CASP)
Critical Appraisal Skills Programme (CASP) use checklists with the aim of helping individuals to develop critiquing skills to make sense of research evidence and bridge the theory–practice gap (CASP, 2006). CASP has

Table 3.4 Quality assessment tool.

Code	Author (year) and country	Aims clear?	Participants appropriate for question?	Design appropriate for aims and theoretical perspective?	Methods appropriate for design?	Sample size and sampling justified?	Does the data analysis fit with the chosen methodology?	Reflexivity present?	Study ethical?	Do the data presented justify the findings?	Is the context described sufficiently?	Is there sufficient evidence of rigour?	Include?

Quality key and rating:

Comments:

Table 3.5 ABCD grading system (A–, A, A+), (B–, B, B+), (C–, C, C+), (D–, D, D+).

Grade	Comments
A	No, or few flaws. The study credibility, transferability, dependability and confirmability are high
B	Some flaws, unlikely to affect the credibility, transferability, dependability and/or confirmability of the study
C	Some flaws that may affect the credibility, transferability, dependability and/or confirmability of the study
D	Significant flaws that are very likely to affect the credibility, transferability, dependability and/or confirmability of the study

developed several useful appraisal tools to help researchers, health professionals and students to critique different research methodologies and theoretical perspectives (CASP, 2006). The tools make use of a number of questions: three general questions and then 10, 11 or 12 more specific questions. This includes two screening questions and if the answer is yes to these questions then eight to ten more detailed questions can be answered to assist to critique research papers.

CASP appraisal tools include:

* systematic reviews;
* randomised controlled trials (RCTs);
* qualitative studies;
* economic evaluation studies;
* cohort studies;
* case control studies;
* diagnostic test studies.

CASP appraisal tools can be used for your own personal development and for a non-profit-making activity. Remember, you will need to reference the source of information. For further information, see weblink http://www.phru.nhs.uk/Pages/PHD/resources.htm.

In addition, the Centre for Evidence-Based Medicine (CEBM) has some critical appraisal sheets for systematic reviews and RCTs that you may find helpful. For further information, see weblink http://www.cebm.net/index.aspx?o=1157.

Table 3.6 details a structured process which has been developed to help you critically appraise a quantitative study. It is similar in some respects to the structured process developed to critically appraise a qualitative research paper; however there is variation in the questions to address a quantitative approach and design. See Box 3.1.

Hierarchy of evidence

The introduction of evidence-based medicine, which evolved to become evidence-based practice, has meant that there has been a tendency to see

Table 3.6 Critiquing a quantitative research paper.

The study	Questions
Publication	Do you think the journal is suitable? Is it midwifery specific? Is the study in date, i.e. from the completion of the study to publication, no longer than 3 years?
Title	Does the title clearly state the type of study, i.e. a RCT, and are the subject and population described?
Abstract	Does it summarise the paper content sufficiently? Is the abstract structured or unstructured? If structured, does it include a short introduction, aim, methods, findings, conclusions and implications? Does the title capture the reader's attention? The length of the abstract is usually 250– 300 words; does it meet this requirement?
Author/s	Who are the authors? Are their qualifications, past publications or current posts detailed in the article and do they give them the credentials to conduct this research?
Funding	How has the study been funded? Could there be a conflict of interest, i.e. commercial funding?
Introduction	Does it provide a contextual focus (background) for the research? Does it give a clear rationale of why the research study was investigated?
Literature review	Is the literature up-to-date? (This usually refers to a 5-year window, however landmark studies in the subject area are acceptable) Has the most recent research evidence been reviewed to provide a balanced argument to either support or challenge the proposed research? Does the research evidence represent a hierarchy of evidence, systematic reviews, RCTs, etc ...? Has the review identified a gap in knowledge, i.e. no research or inconclusive evidence? Has the review clearly identified the need for this study? Has any research been omitted from the literature review discussion? (When conducting a research critique, you should perform your own literature search to reach this conclusion) Does the review make sense?
Methodology	Does it state that a quantitative paradigm has been followed and which quantitative approach has been used? (e.g. experimental, observational) Has the research hypothesis, question, aim or outcomes been clearly stated? Does it describe the research methodology? (e.g. RCT, survey) Are the descriptions of and why the research methodology is utilised understandable to you? Have the authors clearly rationalised why this methodology is appropriate, as opposed to others?
Sample and setting	Is the sample representative of the study population? Is the type of sampling clearly stated? (e.g. random, simple, stratified) Was there a sample size calculation carried out? (i.e. power calculation) Are inclusion/exclusion criteria explained and therefore do you understand why this sample needs to be 'like for like' as possible Is the setting where the study was undertaken described?

Table 3.6 *Continued*

The study	Questions
Method/data collection	Was the most appropriate research method chosen? Were confounding variables controlled for? If, experimental research, were groups comparable? Was a pilot study undertaken to test the study design? Which method of data collection was utilised? Is it clearly explained? Does it match the research methodology? (Usually a structured questionnaire or structured interview)
Data management	Are the procedures for managing the collected data described? Have statistical software packages used for this purpose? Was any coding and cross-checking of data discussed?
Data analysis	Is the data analysis method clearly explained? Have descriptive and inferential statistics been used? Has a statistician been consulted? Has all relevant statistical data been included?
Ethical considerations	Does it state that ethical approval has been gained? Does it state that informed consent was gained from the participants? Have ethical issues been adequately addressed? Has the research governance of the study been explained?
Findings	What are the findings? Do they answer the research hypothesis or question? Are the findings valid and relevant? Are tables, graphs and charts clear and understandable? Do the findings make sense? Are the findings generalisible?
Discussion	Does the discussion highlight the findings and link them to other studies on the same subject? Does the discussion stress the significance or not of the study's findings? Are any limitations referred to? Do you consider there were limitations to this study? Do you consider that the authors have given a true representation of the findings of their study?
Conclusion	Does the conclusion identify the key findings and discussion points? Do the authors make any recommendations for practice or further research?

'evidence' in terms of quantitative research and systematic reviews, and RCTs have been classified as the best levels of evidence. Quality of research evidence is judged and graded by classification systems and RCTs are often referred to as the 'gold standard' and classified very highly (Jahad, 2000). Although RCTs are considered to be the best of all research methods, they are not a panacea to answer all research questions. RCTs are, nevertheless, the most suitable research method to answer questions related to the effects of treatments or interventions in healthcare.

Box 3.1 Checklist for quantitative research – 10 points to remember!

Quantitative research should include:

1. a clear statement of the problem;
2. a referenced background;
3. ethical and research governance considerations;
4. the research approach and methodology;
5. pilot study;
6. details of target population and sample size;
7. data collection techniques and analysis;
8. results and limitations;
9. discussion;
10. recommendations.

Table 3.7 Classification levels.

Classification	Comments
Ia	Evidence obtained from meta-analysis of randomised controlled trials
Ib	Evidence obtained from at least one randomised controlled trial
IIa	Evidence obtained format least one well designed controlled study without randomisation
IIb	Evidence obtained from at least one other type of well designed quasi-experimental study
III	Evidence obtained from well designed non-experimental descriptive studies, such as comparative studies, correlation studies and case studies
IV	Evidence obtained from expert committee reports or opinions and/or clinical experience of respected authorities

In the 1990s, simple grading systems were introduced to help grade evidence to assist in the development of clinical guidelines. An example of this is one that was used by the NHS Executive in the UK. This involved grading evidence using an ABC category system:

A Randomised controlled trials
B Other robust experimental or observational studies
C More limited evidence but the advice relies on expert opinion and has the endorsement of respected authorities

An A score was graded as the highest level of evidence and C as the lowest form of evidence (Mann, 1996).

Grading systems were further developed to take into consideration the different levels of evidence provided by quantitative research studies and evidence from experts and clinical experience of respected authorities. A useful grading system that originated from the US Agency for Health Care Policy and Research and is used by the RCOG clinical green top guidelines. See Tables 3.7 and 3.8.

Table 3.8 Grades of recommendations.

Grade	Comments
A	Requires at least one randomised controlled trial as part of a body of literature of overall good quality and consistency addressing the specific recommendation (Evidence levels 1a, 1b)
B	Requires the availability of well controlled clinical studies but no randomised clinical trials on the topic of recommendations (Evidence levels IIa, IIb, III)
C	Requires evidence obtained from expert committee reports or opinions and/or clinical experiences of respected authorities. Indicates an absence of directly applicable clinical studies of good quality (Evidence level IV)

Good practice point (GPP)

✓	Recommended best practice based on the clinical experience of the guideline development group

Grading evidence is continuing to evolve and the specific focus on study design has limitations, as other factors can influence the quality of evidence. The Grading of Recommendations Assessment, Development and Evaluation (GRADE) Working Group has been developing a new approach to grading evidence that moves away from initial reliance on study design to consider the overall quality of evidence. For further information, see weblink http:// www.gradeworkinggroup.org/.

There is a need to balance evidence, clinical expertise and the preferences of women and their families when planning and giving midwifery care. Sometimes, research evidence is not available to answer a question about the most effective care and, as a result, consensus of opinions is sought from experts in our profession and service users. Knowledge, attitudes, views, behaviour, and what is acceptable and accessible can all contribute to recommendations of care and help develop clinical guidelines.

This indicates that all sources of knowledge and both quantitative and qualitative research evidence need to be considered when planning and giving care. The authors remember reading an article written by Walsh (1996) where he described how evidence-based guidelines for the care of women in labour were developed from evidence collected from quantitative and qualitative research. The Cochrane Database of systematic reviews and register of controlled trials provided quantitative evidence of clinical effectiveness but ethnographic and grounded theory studies provided insights of the views and needs of service users; interestingly, many women wanted their partners to be included in their care. Today, this is a topical area of interest and one of the authors is involved in research exploring the experiences of fathers in maternity care (Steen *et al.*, 2008). See weblink http:// chesterrep.openrepository.com/cdr/handle/10034/48457.

Refining your research question

You may find at this stage that you may need to refine your research question as it may have already been answered effectively or to some extent. If the research question has been answered to some extent you could either repeat the research study to confirm or refute the claims made or you may want to ask something similar to cover a different aspect of your chosen topic of interest. You may have also identified some evidence but when you have critiqued this evidence, it is weak, or was inadequately undertaken and has recognisable flaws; so you may want to repeat the research and improve the study design.

Differences between qualitative and quantitative research

Differences between the naturalistic and positivist paradigms are characterised by their underlying philosophical perspectives. These are namely the ontological (nature of reality) and the epistemological (theory of knowledge). When embarking on research the *'conceptual phase'* that Rees (2003) describes will determine your research paradigm and a qualitative or quantitative approach will be influenced by what you want to know and then how you will find the answers.

Qualitative and quantitative approaches help to structure the type of knowledge that needs to be acquired and, as explained earlier in Chapter 1, different research methods are aligned to the different approaches. To make clearer and reiterate the information written in Chapter 1, a flowchart has been designed to show the research methods associated with the qualitative and quantitative approaches (Figure 3.1).

Different perspectives, such as feminist and applied research (evaluation and action research) can use both qualitative and quantitative approaches to find evidence. When undertaking feminist research, a researcher needs to consider the feminist perspective and the most appropriate research methodology that will answer the research question and meet the study aim and objectives. Applied research can also use both approaches to test or discover the effectiveness or impact of a phenomenon.

Generally, validity and reliability mainly refer to a quantitative research approach as they relate to consistency of measurement and effectiveness of tools and techniques (Bryman, 2008). Credibility and trustworthiness mainly refer to a qualitative research approach as they relate to openness and honesty when interpreting data (Cutler, 2004).

Both qualitative and quantitative research approaches can be used in the same study and some researchers use what is referred to as a mixed methods approach. This can be beneficial when the research needs to investigate and explore a phenomenon. An example of this could be where participants are asked to participate in a focus group interview or one-to-one interviews prior to the undertaking of an RCT or survey (Box 3.2).

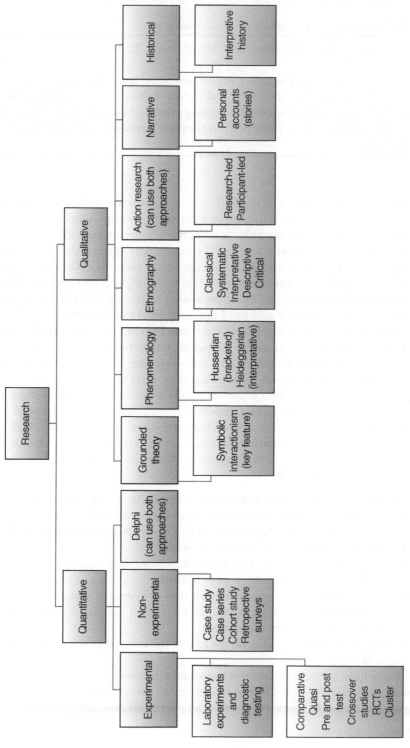

Figure 3.1 Research approaches and methods.

Box 3.2 An example of mixed methods used in a research study.

The Alleviating Perineal Trauma: APT Study (Steen, 2004).

This study carried out laboratory experiments and used focus group interview, randomised controlled trial and survey methods. All methods provided valuable information for the development and evaluation of a newly designed cooling device (femepad) to alleviate perineal trauma following childbirth.

The quantitative aspects of the RCT record measurable outcomes but this has limitations; asking the participants their views or experiences in a focus group setting or on a one-to-one basis will give a deeper insight into an aspect of the outcomes which could be around the care they received, or an opportunity to explore their views and feelings about their involvement in the actual trial itself. Using mixed methods can reveal aspects and concepts that are important to the outcomes being measured (quantitatively) but were not identified by this approach and need (qualitatively) exploring further.

To reiterate what has already been mentioned in Chapter 1, the **qualitative approach** uses methods to gather knowledge that focuses on experiences, thoughts, feelings and behaviour, and acknowledges the use of subjectivity (Davies, 2007). Its overall aim is to understand, from the perspective of participants, the meaning of their experiences (Robinson, 2002) The **quantitative approach** uses methods to gather empirical knowledge and focuses on facts, figures and experiments, and acknowledges the use of objectivity (Begley, 2008). Its overall aim is to produce data that can be '*counted, measured, weighed, enumerated and so manipulated and compared mathematically*' (Grix, 2004, p. 173).

The qualitative approach:

* relies on transforming information from observations, reports and recording the data in the form of the written word (not numbers);
* taped interviews get transformed into transcripts, observations get recorded in field notes, pictures get described in words;
* there is a vast difference in the time it takes to analyse results;
* deals with meanings or patterns of behaviour;
* relies on a detailed and intricate description of events or people;
* exhibits a preference for seeing things in context and for stressing how things are related and interdependent;
* tends to place great emphasis on the role of the researcher in the 'construction of the data';
* there is little use of standardised research instruments;
* recognises the researcher as the crucial 'measurement device';
* theories can be developed and tested as part of an on-going process.

The quantitative approach:

- transforms what is observed, reported or recorded into 'quantifiable' units;
- uses numerical data as the input and statistical procedures;
- numbers are well suited to the kinds of comparisons and correlations required for analysis;
- focuses on specific factors to study them in relation to specific other factors to understand their working and their effect;
- a key feature is the precision with which research designs are established at the outset of the study;
- hypothesis establishes exactly the nature of the research question;
- there is a specific sample;
- uses both experimental and non-experimental methods;
- produces numerical data that are objective and exist independently of the researcher;
- uses validated research tools to assist to achieve this;
- data accurately reflect the event itself.

Table 3.9 summarises the differences between qualitative and quantitative approaches. Box 3.3 contains a checklist of 10 features that can be either

Table 3.9 Qualitative and quantitative approaches.

Qualitative approaches are associated with:	Quantitative approaches are associated with:
Words as the unit of analysis	Numbers as the unit of analysis
Description	Analysis
Small scale	Large scale
A holistic perspective	A specific focus
Researcher involvement	Researcher detachment
An emergent research design	Predetermined research design

Box 3.3 Checklist – qualitative or quantitative?

Circle your answer: **Qualitative** or **Quantitative**

1. Uses data to test a theory   **Qualitative** or **Quantitative**
2. Provides insights and understandings   **Qualitative** or **Quantitative**
3. Uses defined questions to collect   **Qualitative** or **Quantitative**
   precise answers
4. Theories emerge from the data   **Qualitative** or **Quantitative**
5. Non-experimental design   **Qualitative** or **Quantitative**
6. Uses unstructured interviews   **Qualitative** or **Quantitative**
7. Uses a large representative sample   **Qualitative** or **Quantitative**
8. Collects detailed ranked information   **Qualitative** or **Quantitative**
   about participants' attitudes
9. Uses random sampling   **Qualitative** or **Quantitative**
10. Makes inferences to the total   **Qualitative** or **Quantitative**
   population

qualitative or quantitative which you can use to test your knowledge and understanding so far.

Summary

This chapter has covered how to critique research evidence. In recent years, the importance of evidence-based practice has been recognised and critical appraisal is important. It is essential that midwives and students know how to assess and evaluate evidence effectively as this will impact upon their practice. This chapter has, therefore, highlighted some useful critiquing tools available for midwives and students to assess the quality of research studies. The information presented gives an insight into how midwives and students need to undertake critiquing research evidence in a structured and systematic way. Midwives and students need to be very clear about the differences between qualitative and quantitative approaches and methods. For this reason a section in this chapter that describes and discusses the characteristics and differences between qualitative and quantitative approaches and methods has been included. Critiquing both qualitative and quantitative research has been individually discussed and explored. Specific tools to critique the two different research approaches has been included. Research evidence and how this is classified in levels of quality by using structured hierarchy of evidence tools has been included to assist midwives and students to interpret the evidence.

It is envisaged that midwives and students will have gained an understanding of the importance of critiquing evidence. They will have developed some knowledge and skills by reading and working through examples in this chapter. The critiquing tools and techniques will assist midwives and students methodically to critique a published piece of research and evaluate the importance of this research. A structured and systematic critiquing approach helps to draw conclusions as to whether research has made an overall contribution to the body of midwifery knowledge. New knowledge is important as it can influence midwifery care and practice which must be based on the best available evidence. Gathering evidence involves using different data collection tools and the next chapter gives an insight into data collection tools and techniques.

Answers to Box 3.3

1. Quantitative, 2. Qualitative, 3. Qualitative, 4. Quantitative, 5. Quantitative, 6. Qualitative, 7. Quantitative, 8. Quantitative, 9. Quantitative, 10. Quantitative.

PART II

II Undertaking research

4 Data collection techniques

Introduction to data collection

This chapter will focus on how to collect data. It will explore and discuss both qualitative and quantitative data collection techniques. In particular, this chapter will guide midwives and students on how to undertake a research interview and how to design a questionnaire, as these two data collection techniques are very common and it is highly likely that midwives and students will choose one of these techniques when starting to undertake research.

Aim

The aim of this chapter is to enable readers to explore the different types of data collection techniques that are available for midwives and students when undertaking research.

Learning outcomes

By the end of this chapter midwives and students:

- will be able to recognise different data collection methods;
- will have gained knowledge and skills of qualitative data collection techniques;
- will have gained knowledge and skills of quantitative data collection techniques;
- will be able to use these techniques to assist them to collect both qualitative and quantitative data;
- will have gained an insight into how to design a questionnaire;
- will have gained an insight into how to design an interview schedule on a midwifery topic of their choice.

Introduction to data collection techniques

Data can be collected using both qualitative and quantitative methods. Usually, researchers chose one of these methods depending on what research

The Handbook of Midwifery Research, First Edition. Mary Steen and Taniya Roberts.
© 2011 Mary Steen and Taniya Roberts. Published 2011 by Blackwell Publishing Ltd.

question they want to ask and which is the most appropriate. However, more and more researchers are recognising the value of mixed methods and may use both methods in a study. Generally, data collection involves some form of observing, assessing, measuring, recording, analysing, interpreting and reporting. In midwifery, it will usually involve the actions and behaviour of women, their babies and families, or the actions and behaviour of midwives and students themselves. Research is undertaken in educational, clinical and home settings and data collected are related to either exploring views and experiences or testing out treatments/interventions and evaluating ways of working. The data collected can be prospective (on-going) or retrospective (looking back).

Data collection for both the qualitative and quantitative approaches can appear to be quite similar, but the application and retrieval of information does differ. An example is conducting an interview. Both approaches can utilise this data collection tool: following a qualitative approach, unstructured and semi-structured interviews are favoured, whereas the quantitative approach utilises a highly structured format. This chapter will describe the use of the different data collection methods for the different approaches.

Things to consider include:

- How do I collect the data?
- What do I need to know and why?
- What shall I do with it?
- How much time do I have?
- Would another researcher be able to get similar responses?

Limiting study bias

Recognising and limiting the potential for bias is an important aspect that researchers have to consider. Before any data collection technique is designed, it is necessary to take into account any issue or aspect that might affect the study design and outcomes to be measured. The findings from a research study should be as free from bias as possible. This will increase the credibility and trustworthiness of qualitative studies and the validity and reliability of quantitative studies.

Researcher bias

A researcher needs to be aware of the influences that their own beliefs and views can have on the research topic and how this can affect the research design and study (Baker, 2006). It is important for a researcher to be reflective and, at regular intervals, consider how their beliefs and views are influencing the study in order to reduce personal bias (Kingdon, 2005).

Sample size

Qualitative and quantitative approaches will require different sample sizes. Guidelines for determining qualitative sample size are limited. Collection of qualitative data often involves large quantities of written text from one-to-one interviews or focus group interviews; this approach involves in-depth exploration of the data which can be gathered from a relatively small number of participants. At the outset, a sample size for qualitative studies may not be decided. When a 'saturation point' is reached (the data is producing no emerging new themes or concepts), this will influence the sample size and indicate that the researcher should discontinue. Guest *et al.* (2006) used data from a study which involved 60 women from West Africa who had consented to an in-depth interview. The researchers systematically documented the degree of data saturation and variability over the course of the thematic analysis undertaken. They found that saturation occurred within the first 12 interviews but basic elements for meta-themes were evident as early as six interviews and variability with the data followed similar patterns.

In contrast, sample sizes for quantitative studies are usually determined by statistical estimates. This is calculated by the number of participants required to be involved to demonstrate that the findings were due to the effect of the intervention/treatment investigated in the trial and not due to chance.

Types of quantitative sampling include:

- random sampling:
    ○ simple – all have equal chance of inclusion;
    ○ stratified – uses certain characteristics or subgroups;
- cluster: uses several sites and can recruit in stages;
- systematic: uses a way to identify, e.g. every third person on a list.

Note: everyone has a known chance of selection.

Qualitative data collection techniques

Qualitative sampling

Researchers would find it difficult, time consuming and extremely expensive to conduct research on the population and that is why determining the sample, i.e. a group, culture or organisation that represents the population, is a very important aspect of the research design. A sample refers to a group of people who represent the aim of the research (Griffiths, 2009). For example if the aim of the study is find out how first-time mothers have experienced breastfeeding support from student midwives, then a sample of first-time mothers, who have received breastfeeding support from student midwives, would need to be recruited. Strict inclusion and exclusion criteria are required in any research study to set the parameters of who should be included or not (Table 4.1). This does require careful consideration in the design phase of the study.

The type of sampling used for qualitative research comes under the term of non-probability sampling, which means that the chance of any individual being selected is not known. Its purpose is not to generalise the findings but to identify certain relevant issues (Parahoo, 2006). The following types of

Table 4.1 Example of inclusion and exclusion criteria.

Inclusion criteria	Exclusion criteria
First-time mothers who have breastfed for at least 1 month and received support from at least one student midwife	Bottlefeeding mothers Breastfeeding mothers who did not receive support from student midwives Mothers who have breastfed before Mothers who have breastfed for less than 1 month

sampling are the most common to qualitative research. A purposive sample is known to possess key characteristics which can best inform the research, therefore the participants are essentially handpicked to take part (Denscombe, 2003). In snowball sampling the researcher identifies some individuals who possess the necessary characteristics/experiences and then asks these to suggest others who may be willing to participate. With convenience sampling the researcher selects the most easily accessible people from the population (Davies, 2007). Open sampling requires the researcher to be open to interviewing any participant and observing any events as important issues emerge. Theoretical sampling takes over when the sample is decided by the emerging theory (information/categories) (Charmaz, 2006).

Sample size in qualitative research is usually small, with no specific sample numbers planned in the design stage of the study. The sample size therefore becomes dependent on the information gathered from data collection. In qualitative research when no new information is determined from the participants the term used is called saturation (Cluett & Bluff, 2006). When saturation is reached the sample size is complete and data collection is finalised.

When the participants have been selected, the following procedures must be adhered to before data collection commences. There must be informed consent, confidentiality must be ensured, permission has to be obtained to audio-tape interviews and publish results, and finally a time and place have to be agreed for data collection (Mapp, 2008).

Phenomenology and sampling

In phenomenology, purposive sampling is used, selecting individuals who will have knowledge of the phenomena concerned; this therefore allows an understanding of the lived experience. The sample can be representative of participants who are living the experience or those that have previously lived it (Cohen, 2002), e.g. women's experiences of obstetric emergencies (Mapp & Hudson, 2005).

As the intention is not to generalise the findings, there is no requirement for large numbers of participants. Carpenter (1999) suggests that the sample size in phenomenological research should be small, in order that every experience can be examined in depth. Using this research methodology can make prediction of the sample size difficult, as sampling should continue until saturation is reached, i.e. no new categories occur during data collection (Macnee, 2004).

Ethnography and sampling

In any ethnographic study, Hegelund (2005, p. 651) suggests that the first step is to define the *'object of study'*. When this has been determined, consent given to the environment and participants and ethical approval gained (Donovan, 2006), data collection can proceed, beginning with observation. The sampling usually associated with this research methodology is purposive, which requires the researcher to choose a specific group and setting to be studied (Price & Johnson, 2006). There is a further sub-group to the sample, which originates from within the participants being studied. This group is interviewed to determine the meaning of the behaviour observed (Brink & Edgecombe, 2003). This allows for an understanding of why people behave in a certain way in certain circumstances.

Grounded theory and sampling

Initially sampling can take the form of open sampling, where the researcher is at liberty to interview any participant, observe any event or examine any documents (Bluff, 2006). As the information is collated and analysed the sampling changes to one of theoretical sampling, whereby the sample is determined by any issues which have emerged and becomes more focused on the individuals or phenomena to be studied (Burns & Grove, 2005).

Qualitative data collection tools

There are many different data collection tools/methods/techniques available, that can be used within the qualitative approach. Examples are observation, one-to-one interviews, focus group interviews, examining written texts (books, transcripts, historical facts, songs, poetry) story telling (oral narratives), video and films. Specific tools are, however, aligned to specific methodology, e.g. ethnography and observation. Information within this chapter will demonstrate the use and purpose of some of these data collection methods, however, an explanation is needed on the subject of trustworthiness, which is an essential element to qualitative data collection.

Trustworthiness

'Trustworthiness is about ensuring that qualitative research represents the truth' (Morgan, 2004, p. 61); it is an essential component in qualitative data collection. In 1985, Lincoln and Guba suggested a framework of four criteria, credibility, dependability, confirmability and tranferability, to determine the truthfulness of qualitative research. Their aim was to provide a structure to match the quantitative approach's key requirements of internal validity, reliability, objectivity and external validity. In 1994 they added aunthenticity, to strengthen the rigour of this process (Polit & Beck, 2008, p. 492). Box 4.1 gives an explanation of the components of determining trustworthiness.

Box 4.1 Components of trustworthiness.

- **Credibility** – refers to confidence in the truth of the data (validity) and interpretations of them.
- **Dependability** – refers to the stability (reliability) of data over time and conditions. It calls for an audit trail, the explicit steps the researcher has taken throughout the research study.
- **Confirmability** – refers to the data being true representations of the information that the participants have provided (not influenced/biased by the researcher).
- **Transferability** – refers to the extent to which the study's findings can be transferred to other settings or groups (generalisability).
- **Authenticity** – refers to the extent to which researchers fairly and faithfully show a range of different realities.

(Polit & Beck, 2008, p. 492–493)

A qualitative study should therefore be able to demonstrate the components of trustworthiness to ensure its integrity.

Ethnography and data collection – observation

Generally there are perceived to be two types of observation used in this research methodology. Rees (2003) suggests they are participant or non-participant observation, with the researcher being the major research tool for data collection. There is, however, a body of opinion which suggests that there are four types of observation in ethnography. Donovan (2006, p. 137) suggests that these are 'complete participant, participant-as-observer, observer-as-participant and complete observer'. Brink and Edgecombe (2003, p. 1029) believe that the signature of ethnography is 'the use of participant observation', and this is characterised by the researcher becoming submerged within the culture, and subsequent 'day to day lives' of those who are being studied (Grix, 2004, p. 166).

In participant observation the researcher endeavours to become part of the culture by being in the field, as opposed to a more detached stance as in non-participant observation (Denscombe, 2003). The intention of the non-participant observer is, therefore, to record observations within the setting that is being studied, but without any interaction (Roberts, 2009). In participant observation, there are circumstances in which the researcher's role may not be disclosed to participants, despite the inherent ethical difficulties (Rugg & Petre, 2007). However, in order that the researcher can discuss what has been observed with the participants, Davies (2007) recommends that their research role is revealed. For both the participant and non-participant researcher everything that is seen and heard is recorded/noted in the field notes and can potentially become the starting points for any in-depth interviews which may follow (Roberts, 2009).

There are advantages and disadvantages to the use of either type of observation. The advantages of the participant observation are that the researcher is part of the situation and is more aware of morale, apathy and goodwill, and the researcher might also be seen as having credibility by those being observed (Davies, 2007). The disadvantages of participant observation are that the researcher can have potential difficulties recording observations in a busy clinical area (Parahoo, 2006) and participants may view the researcher as a threat or 'mole', which can adversely affect the accuracy of the observation. For non-participant observation, the researcher can follow a more structured plan of observation. The potential difficulties are that the observer might be conspicuous, thereby directly affecting what is observed and those being observed may try and interact with the observer (Donovan, 2006). Carthey (2003) suggests that two observers are often necessary to guard against possible bias.

Both types of observation can prove to be very time consuming, and prolonged observation is the ideal. Williams (2008) suggests that typically this time can range from 6 to 18 months or longer. There can, however, be a limit to the amount of time for observation and a criticism of ethnographic healthcare research has been that some studies have not been developed to the extent that they could have been (Holloway & Todres, 2006).

It is possible for data collection methods to also incorporate photography and the use of video cameras (Pink, 2007). Ethnographers are also open to visual analysis of any artefacts, i.e. any objects relating to the subject of the research or document witnessed within the environment under study (Lindsay, 2007), for example, the noticeboards in the clinical area.

It is important that collecting information from observations is conducted in a systematic manner (Parahoo, 2006), otherwise field notes may not be usable. Davies (2007) recommends that the researcher has a system worked out prior to data collection as to how the observations will be recorded, i.e. field notes in a diary, an audio recorder.

When conducting this type of research, midwifery researchers must always consider their potential actions if they were to observe unsafe practice and ensure they have developed a strategy in line with the NMC Code (NMC, 2008).

It is possible that during the data collection by observation, the researcher may not understand what has been seen, and they should therefore seek clarification from members of the group or culture to explain it to them (John & Parsons, 2006; Price & Johnson, 2006).

Further data are collected by the use of audio-taped semi-structured interviews (van Teijlingen & Ireland, 2003). The actual length of the interviews is dictated by the process of saturation, i.e. when no new data are revealed (Sim & Wright, 2000).

It is important to note that the terms 'emic and 'etic' are commonly used in ethnography. The interviews provide the 'emic', which is the insiders' perceptions, to enable the researcher to uncover knowledge of why people behave in a specific way. The 'etic' is the alternative perspective, which refers to the researcher's attempts to make sense of what has been observed without the group's explanations (Rees, 2003).

Limitations
In using this research methodology there are potential limitations, and the Hawthorne effect is one that researchers new to ethnography should be aware of. It reasons that if people are aware that they are being observed, they may change their behaviour (Rees, 2003). There is a suggestion however, that this has been over-emphasised, and that most professional groups are just too busy to keep up behaviour which is different to their norm (Mulhall, 2003).

A further potential problem with this type of research is that it can be difficult for the researcher not to become too immersed, and too subjective, whilst in the field (Parahoo, 2006); or *'going native'* and straying from the role of observer (Barbour, 2008). This is further acknowledged by Rees (2003) who suggests that midwifery researchers should acquire the role of the *'enquiring stranger'*, as opposed to interpreting what they are observing by means of their own midwifery knowledge.

Grounded theory data collection and data analysis
What stands out in this research methodology and makes it different to others is that data collection and analysis are linked from the beginning of the research, proceed in parallel and interact continuously (Strauss & Corbin 1998). The researchers therefore start with an area of interest, collect data and allow relevant ideas to develop, ideally without preconceived theories (Grix, 2004). This allows for the emergence of new theories and alternative perspectives rather than following previously developed ideas (Roberts, 2008).

Data collection can take the format of interviews, narratives, field notes and observations. However, Polit and Beck (2008) suggest that interviews are the most commonly used; they are audio-taped and transcribed verbatim.

Interviews
Undertaking a research interview will be further explained later in this chapter, the following information details how interviews are conducted following the qualitative approach and with particular reference to phenomenology, ethnography and grounded theory.

One-to-one interviews
There are different types of individual research interviews, from low/ unstructured to semi-structured to highly structured formats. The aim of formulating an interview following the qualitative approach (exploring thoughts, feelings, beliefs and experiences) is to gain clarity and understanding from the perspectives of the participants. Conversely, a highly structured interview could potentially reveal information from the perspective of the researcher. This means that low/unstructured to semi-structured interviews

meet the requirements of the qualitative research approach. Unstructured interviewing can also be used for narrative research (Jones, 2004).

Phenomenology and the research interview – unstructured
In both Husserlian and Heidergerrian phenomenology research the optimum method for data collection is by unstructured one-to-one interviews (Webb, 2003; Carpenter, 2007; Mapp, 2008). To remain as true to this type of research methodology as possible it is feasible that following an unstructured approach will yield enough responses that encapsulate the whole experience (Mapp & Hudson, 2005) from the perspectives of the participants, rather than that of the researchers.

The unstructured interview should start with a question such as 'tell me about your experience'. Ideally, no other questions should be asked, however a researcher may sense that the interviewee has more to tell and Gillham (2005, p. 32-33) recommends the use of probes as a *'form of responsive encouragement; to help them expand or clarify or develop their account'*. The researcher may say 'I'm not sure I've quite got that', so the interviewee clarifies or explains or expands on what they are describing from their perspective. Using phrases such as 'take your time', can reassure participants and aid the flow of the interview (Jones, 2004, p. 43).

The technique of phenomenological interviewing following a Husserlian approach differs to the Heidegerrian approach in that it requires the researcher to put aside her preconceived ideas regarding the subject of the interview prior to data collection. The researcher is therefore required to follow the process of bracketing, i.e. setting aside prejudgement (Mapp, 2008).

A distinct advantage of using interviews is that they can draw from the interviewee a vivid picture of the experience, which leads to clarity and understanding of shared meanings (Sorrell & Redmond, 1995). This element fulfills the aim of Husserlian phenomenology, which is to describe people's experiences of phenomena and how they understand them. This, however, can only be achieved if the participants are not influenced by the researcher (Mapp, 2008).

Moustakas (1994) suggests that the interview begins with a social conversation with the intention of creating a relaxed and trusting atmosphere. The researcher can then suggest that the interviewee takes a few moments to focus on the experience fully, before the interview commences. By the researcher adopting a supportive and trustworthy approach, the participants are encouraged to describe their experiences without bias until data saturation is achieved (Mapp, 2008).

The length of a phenomenological interview is guided by the process of saturation, i.e. when the narratives become repetitive and no new data is revealed. Data saturation can range from 30 to 120 minutes (Berg & Dahlberg, 1998; Lundqvist *et al.*, 2002).

In the main, phenomenological interviews are audio-taped because they can provide a rich source of data, which can be analysed after the interview.

It is entirely possible that nuances of description can easily be missed if the interviewer is handwriting the notes of the interview whilst it is in progress. The researcher should also have the facility to make notes once the tape recording has finished, because at this time it is not unusual for participants to provide more information (Mapp, 2008).

There are certain disadvantages in using this data collection method. It can, for instance, be time consuming, is labour intensive, costly and requires interviewers to be highly skilled in this technique (Parahoo, 2006). Interviewees can also potentially become very distressed and agitated during the interview, depending upon the subject matter (Rees, 2003). Generally, though, midwives are well equipped with the necessary communication skills to conduct interviews using a phenomenological approach (Robinson, 2006).

The location for the interview is usually in an environment where the participant spends their time (Mapp, 2008). There should be an opportunity, however, for the participant to be interviewed away from their home environment, in a private room free from interruptions if they desire. Funding, therefore, has to be a consideration in the research design phase of the study so that there is the availability of monies for the cost of transport or childcare to enable participants to take part in a research study.

Ethnography and grounded theory interviews – semi-structured
Ethnography and grounded theory interviews favour the semi-structured approach. In ethnographic research the researcher wants to gather information to understand what has been observed. In grounded theory the interview is used to try and understand an emerging concept or reality (Charmaz, 2006). The researcher therefore wants to gain clarity and understanding from the perspectives of the participants not from their own perspective, which a highly structured interview would potentially reveal.

The types of questions asked in a semi-structured format are usually 'open'. An open-ended question such as 'can you tell me more…can you tell me why?' is hoping to elicit information from the participant's perspective which can lead to the researcher understanding what they have observed (e.g. behaviour observed on a busy delivery suite in ethnography) and developing information (grounded theory). With this type of interview the researcher requires an interview guide – a list of some questions to help guide the interview (Rees, 2003). It is advisable to make notes regarding the interview, e.g. participants' behaviour, new insights, whether there were interruptions.

Group interviews
Group interviews can also be referred to as focus group interviews. Gillham (2005) suggests that they can be used as either data collection for the early stages of an exploratory study or as one of the data collection methods as part of a large empirical study. The structure of a focus group involves a group of people who are asked about a topic or, in some circumstances, just given a topic to discuss. Each group is assigned a facilitator to aid the flow of discus-

sion and ensure everyone has a voice. This person is not necessarily the researcher as the researcher may adversely influence data collection. Facilitating a group and collecting data at the same time can be very difficult. Gillham (2005, p. 62) recommends videoing focus groups as this enables a better analysis of the recorded information, just audio-taping the interview is fraught with difficulties – *'people are slightly better behaved – in the sense of turn-taking – when they know they are being videoed'*.

The size of the group should be no less than six and no more than ten participants and they should have knowledge of, interest in or experience of the topic to be discussed (Macdonald, 2004). The benefits of this type of interviewing are that, amid the group dynamics, it may reveal information/issues about a situation which were not disclosed during individual interviews.

Undertaking a research interview

Introduction
A common data collection tool used when undertaking qualitative research is an interview. Some preparation and practice are required prior to undertaking a research interview. Generally speaking you will have had some life experience of being an interviewee or interviewer on an unstructured basis (Parahoo, 2006). Conversations are the most effective way people can express themselves; feelings, views, attitudes and experiences are discovered and shared. In your personal and professional life you will have asked and answered questions during conversations. However, these are informal and you will all have experienced some formal type of interview such as when you applied for a midwifery student place at university or when applying for a midwifery position upon qualifying. As you will recall this type of interaction is very different from having a general conversation with a friend, family member or colleague. These interviews have a clear agenda and are structured with a specific focus, i.e. are you a suitable candidate?

As a midwife you have frequently carried out interviews, for example when booking a woman for antenatal care which involves asking questions, giving information and discussion. The overall purpose of the booking interview is to obtain information about the health and well-being of the woman, to assess whether she is low or high risk, discuss her pathway of care and her concerns, start to develop a relationship and build trust. This experience should help you to develop research interview skills and techniques.

A research interview also has a specific focus and that is to collect data to answer a research question(s) about a phenomenon of interest. The degree of interaction between the interviewee and interviewer can vary depending on the research approach and type of interview.

Conducting an interview can be an intense and time-consuming process, the interviewer has to become immersed into understanding the situation from the participants' perspective. It is a subjective, not objective process; however, reflexivity needs to be practised. It is important that the researcher has a clear concept of what form the interviews are to take to answer the research question. Equally they should have awareness of the difficulties they may face when conducting the interview both individually and as a group.

Types of interviews

Interviews can be face-to-face, i.e. one-to-one or focus group approach, which usually involves both the researcher and the participant(s) being physically present, i.e. in the same room. However, increasingly now the options of video conferencing facilities and the internet are being used; these alternatives have the benefits of involving international participation and costs can be kept to a minimum (Scholl *et al.*, 2002).

Telephone interviews are also an option and this approach can be less expensive and time consuming when compared with face-to-face interviews; this is something to consider when designing your research study and planning the work and data collection tool. This method is not without its problems, you will have to consider such things as accessibility, availability, confidentiality and phone connection. We would advise if you are considering using this method to use a land line and arrange a convenient time for the participant to be contacted and ideally on their own to reduce the risk of being interrupted and to ensure confidentiality, i.e. not being overheard. There is some evidence that response rates can be lower than when face-to-face interviews are undertaken and participants may become less engaged in the interview process and display dissatisfaction with the length of interview even though it is usually undertaken in less time (Holbrook *et al.*, 2003).

That said, midwifery research has an excellent example to reflect upon where the telephone interview method was successfully used by Sleep and Grant (1988). This survey investigated what midwifery units in the UK offered and advised to relieve perineal pain following childbirth and the findings demonstrated that a range of systemic and localised treatments was available for women to use but evidence to support their effectiveness was limited. See Box 4.2, for a more recent midwifery example.

The telephone interview method appears to be not as popular as face-to-face interviews and this may indicate that researchers and participants prefer physical contact where body language and cues can be read.

Interview format and process

The type of data a researcher wants to gather will influence the interview format and process. The interview format can be basically dichotomised into either a **structured** or **unstructured** format. Saunders *et al.* (2009) describe how interviews may be highly formalised and structured, using standardised questions for each participant, or they may be informal and unstructured. However, how structured and unstructured the interview will be has to be considered. A researcher will need to have some control over the interview format and process and, therefore, there is no such thing as a totally unstruc-

Box 4.2 An example of a midwifery telephone interview.

Mitchell and Williams (2007) used telephone interviews for pragmatic reasons (respondents were from a wide geographical area). The aim of the study was to explore the role of midwife-complementary therapists. Using a semi-structured interview schedule, eight certified midwife-complementary therapists practising within mainstream maternity services were asked their views regarding the contribution complementary therapies might make to supporting normal birth. The telephone interviews were audio-taped and data were subjected to thematic and content analysis. A core theme was identified, being that complementary therapies support normal birth. Four sub-themes were also identified: complementary therapies provide alternatives and reduce medical intervention, empower women and give them confidence, give midwives the opportunity to be 'with woman' and enable the provision of holistic care.

tured interview format (Jones, 1985). If a qualitative research interview is being planned then the nearest thing to an unstructured format would be when the researcher initially introduces a phenomenon to be explored and asks a research question, then leaves the participant to answer this with as little as possible interruption other than minimal encouragers such as, nods, a smile or 'hmms'. It is important to note that interviews can also be used when a quantitative research approach has been adopted but this will involve using a structured predetermined set of questions that will be asked in a consistent and standardised way to all participants.

Generally speaking, researchers will often adopt one of three interview formats ranging from a structured format to something in between (semi-structured) to a limited structure (unstructured). The type of interview, reflects the flexibility a researcher has when undertaking an interview: what type of data are to be collected, whether the process is to be descriptive and making an inference or exploring meaning and trying to understand.

Unstructured interview

An unstructured interview is used when undertaking qualitative research. An open question is asked by the researcher and the participant takes the lead and in general expresses his or her feelings, perceptions, views and experiences on a particular issue. Non-verbal communication is observed, brief notes can be made and prompts are used to help the interview flow. Unstructured interviews can sometimes be difficult to facilitate and therefore a degree of structure is necessary: a participant can be guided to focus on a particular issue and a topic guide maybe helpful. Commonly the interview is tape-recorded with the participant's permission. This interview format fits well with phenomenological, ethnographic and grounded theory research approaches discussed in earlier chapters. See Box 4.3.

Box 4.3 An example of an individual interview guide (Simpson, 2007).

Aims: to explore the inner meaning attributed to expert intrapartum midwifery practice.

1. I want you to think of someone who you regard an expert in intrapartum care. Tell me about your encounters with that person (or a specific encounter that best demonstrates his/her expertise).
   Prompts:

- Tell me about some experiences that you may have had working with him/her.
- What is she/he like as a person?
- What is it that makes her/him different from other midwives?
- What do women think of her/him?
- What do you think her/his midwifery philosophy is?
- How does she/he view/use technology?

Look for issues surrounding:

- intuition;
- courage;
- leadership;
- knowledge/education;
- skills;
- judgement.

If not spontaneously explored by participants ask:

2. How does he/she facilitate or promote normal birth? Can you tell me about any experiences you may have had?
3. Have you worked with him/her in high-risk or emergency situations? Can you tell me about that experience?

Semi-structured interview

Using a semi-structured format allows the researcher to keep some control over the content and process during the interview. An interview schedule is often used by the researcher to prompt and progress the interview steadily which allows a semi-structured format to be used. This in-between format enables data that is both descriptive and exploratory to be collected and analysed. The participants have the opportunity to answer both open and closed questions which allows for some structure of questions and then the option to expand upon the answers. Box 4.4 gives an example which was used in a qualitative midwifery research study undertaken by Steen and Calvert (2007).

Box 4.4 An example of an interview schedule relating to the use of the kit of Homeopathic Remedies for Childbirth.

- Did the use of the kit provide a means to help you cope during childbirth?
- Did you use the kit specifically for pain relief?
- Do you feel the use of the kit of Homeopathic Remedies for Childbirth improved your experience of childbirth?
- What were the positive benefits, if any, of using the kit of Homeopathic Remedies for Childbirth?
- What were the negative aspects, if any, of using the kit of Homeopathic Remedies for Childbirth?
- Did you experience any problems in using the self-administrating kit?
- Were there any symptoms or conditions which were not covered by the remedies available in the kit?
- Did your birth partner become involved in administering remedies?
- What did you feel was the attitude of your birth partner regarding the kit of Homeopathic Remedies for Childbirth?
- What was the attitude of the midwifery and medical staff regarding your use of the kit of Homeopathic Remedies for Childbirth?
- Would you use the kit of Homeopathic Remedies for Childbirth again?
- Would you recommend the kit of Homeopathic Remedies for Childbirth to others?
- Any other comments?

Structured interview

A structured interview involves some form of standardised question format and questions are asked in a systematic and sequential way (Table 4.2). The same questions are asked in the same way to all participants. A standard designed questionnaire could be used by the researcher in an interview but it could also be used during a telephone interview or sent by post to participants to self complete. However, it can be beneficial for the researcher to be present as it encourages and motivates the participant to respond and answer the questions. This approach is useful when large samples are recruited in a survey and quantitative data need to be collected from a target population so comparisons can be made between homogeneous (similar) individuals.

In general, some participants will have reading and writing difficulties and for these in particular a research interview will give a researcher the opportunity to assist them to answer questions and participate in research. Face-to-face interviews offer an opportunity to clarify any misunderstandings and also allow for further explanation if a participant is unclear what the question is asking. Participants need to be able to understand what the question means to enable them to answer truthfully and honestly. How questions are asked is left to the researcher and there maybe occasions when a

Table 4.2 An example of a structured interview schedule – diet and nutrition (Steen, 2010).

	Question	True	or	False
1	The quality of food and not the quantity is the key to a healthy diet during pregnancy			
2	Convenience foods such as pies, biscuits, crisps, cake are high in nutrients			
3	Coffee acts as an anti-nutrient			
4	If pregnant women drink tea with their meals this does not have an effect on iron intake			
5	On average a pregnant woman only needs an extra 200 calories per day in the last trimester			
6	Milk is a rich source of calcium but a poor source of magnesium			
7	Eating a diet rich in calcium and magnesium can help reduce the risk of muscle cramps during pregnancy			
8	A poor fluid intake can be a cause of muscle cramps			
9	Antioxidants are helpful in reducing the likelihood of pre-eclampsia during pregnancy			
10	Women gain on average about 12 kg (28 pounds) during pregnancy			

researcher may have to re-phrase the question so a participant understands. However, be aware that a researcher's presence can introduce bias and participants may be more inclined to give answers that they feel are what the researcher wants to hear. In addition, personal characteristics of the researcher can also influence to some extent how a participant will answer the questions. Cartwright (1986) has highlighted that the gender, age, race and even what a researcher is wearing and their accent can all influence how a participant will respond.

Focus group interview
Focus groups have been widely used to examine people's experiences of ill health and health services (Morgan, 1997). A focus group can instigate one group member to prompt another to contribute and express their views on challenging issues more readily than when individual interviews are undertaken. However, group dynamics have to be considered (Tuckman & Jenson,

1977). Forsyth (1990) describes five stages that may occur within group dynamics, these are forming, storming, norming, performing and adjourning. A researcher will need to guide the group when facilitating a focus group interview; at the outset, clear ground rules, such as not interrupting when someone else is speaking and valuing each other's contributions, are essential. The dynamic interaction of the group can also provide an insight into people's attitudes, perceptions and opinions (Kitzinger, 1994) and dissent between participants can clarify beliefs and reveal underlying assumptions. The focus group data analysis will also seek issues with strong group-to-group validation and *'sensitive moments'* within group interactions that indicated difficult but important issues (Barbour & Kitzinger, 1999). Reliability can be enhanced by identifying issues that are consistent between the focus groups. Deviant cases will be actively sought throughout the analysis and emerging ideas and themes modified in response (Silverman, 1997). See Box 4.5.

Box 4.5 Group interview guide (Simpson, 2007).

Welcome participants to group. Remind about tape-recording and assuring confidentiality.

Concept: expertise
1. What qualities do you think 'expert midwives' have?

   Prompts:

   • What about expertise in the area of normality?
   • and in the area of pathology?
   • and in other areas (please specify)?

Concept: normal birth
2. What does the term normal birth mean to you?

   Prompts:

   • Is normal birth important? Why? Why not?
   • What midwifery practices and treatments are acceptable/not acceptable within the boundaries of normal birth? Why?
   • What medical or anaesthetic activities and treatments are acceptable/ not acceptable within the boundaries of normal birth? Why?
   • What do you think women understand by the term normal birth?

Concept: facilitating normal birth
3. How do midwives facilitate normal birth?

Continued

Prompts:

- Do different ways of organising staff make a difference? How, why?
- Does the place of birth make a difference? How, why?
- Do midwifery or medical practices make a difference? How, why?
- Do the beliefs and philosophies of the attending professionals make a difference? How, why?
- What about the beliefs and philosophies of the woman, her partner, her family?

4. What do you think are the qualities of an expert midwife in the area of normal birth?

This question is a bit more focused than question 1. Please answer this question by thinking about someone you think is an expert in this area, and telling us what is particular about them (without naming them or identifying them to the group).

Prompts:

- demographics (age, years qualified years experienced for example);
- personality;
- skills or beliefs.

Quantitative data collection techniques

Quantitative data collection involves data that can be collected by observation, experiments and research that uses an experimental design such as a randomised controlled trial (RCT) or non-experimental design such as a survey method.

Observation
Observation is a primary method used to collect data and usually involves physical presence. It can be undertaken on a one-to-one basis or within a group and is usually unstructured. It is often used as a supplementary technique and as a precursor to subsequent testing of insights or hypotheses. When experimental research is being undertaken this will involve some form of controlled observation when assessing and collecting data. Some type of structured observation will be used when undertaking a survey or when interviewing.

Hawthorne effect
The Hawthorne effect is a form of reactivity whereby subjects improve an aspect of their behaviour being experimentally measured simply in response to the fact that they are being studied and not in response to any particular experimental manipulation (Leonard, 2008).

Experiments

Experiments involve observing, measuring, testing and recording events. Laboratory experiments can find valuable answers about how to treat diseases and conditions; in medicine great advances have been made during the last 100 years. It is unusual for midwives to carry out experiments whilst undertaking research studies but this may be necessary if a new treatment is being developed. An example of a midwifery-led experiment was the warming and cooling rates of different gel compositions in a laboratory setting undertaken by one of the authors (Steen & Cooper, 1998). These laboratory experiments were undertaken to find the most suitable gel composition to use in a specifically designed 'Maternity Gel Pad' to alleviate perineal trauma. The main aim of the laboratory experiments was to identify the type and concentration of a gel composition that would:

- remain pseudo-plastic over a temperature range of −20°C to +40°C;
- have a high thermal capacity;
- cool quickly when placed in a domestic freezer;
- warm up to external body temperature within 30 minutes when placed on the perineum.

Figures 4.1 and 4.2 show examples of some of the laboratory findings of cooling and warming rates for the most suitable gel composition. These experiments provided valuable information prior to a RCT (Steen *et al.*, 2000). Profiles of controlled cooling and warming rates were observed and therefore the risks of a delay in healing by excessive cooling or exacerbating inflammation by warming were minimised. These laboratory experiments provided scientific evidence as to which gel composition was the most suitable to use.

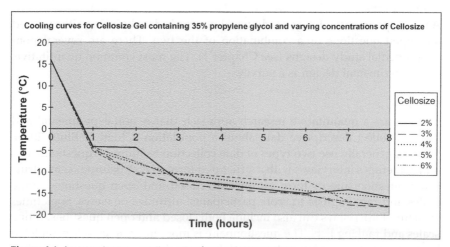

Figure 4.1 An experiment − cooling rates for a gel composition.

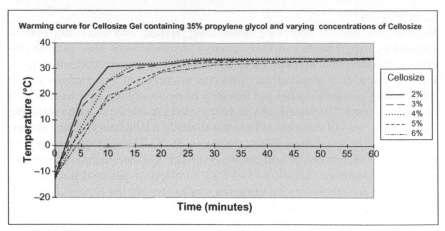

Figure 4.2 An experiment – warming rates for a gel composition.

Observational study

An observational study usually uses data recording sheets and question-naires. Factual information is recorded and can measure all types of data: nominal, ordinal, ratio and interval (see the section in Chapter 6, A basic understanding of statistics).

Experimental design study

An experimental design study usually records data by using closed questions and rating scales in a structured questionnaire or structured interview format but it can also be semi-structured and include some open questions to explore qualitative aspects relating to the subject matter.

Non-experimental design study

A non-experimental design study usually records data by using either closed and open questions or a combination of the two. There are several non-experimental study designs (see Chapter 1). The most common quantitative, non-experimental design is a survey.

Surveys

Surveys are a quantitative research approach that is non-experimental and aims to collect descriptive data about a population (Cluett & Bluff, 2006). Surveys generally use two types of data collection techniques: questionnaires and sometimes interviews with a structured format. A structured/semi-structured questionnaire or form can include closed and open questions, rating scales and ranking lists to score participants' attitudes or views. Sometimes structured interviews can also include both closed and open questions, rating scales and ranking lists. The questionnaire is more likely to be self-completed by the respondents and the interview data is usually recorded by the researcher.

Survey research has evolved over the last decade and more and more on-line surveys are being introduced as opposed to the more commonly used postal survey.

Undertaking a survey involves 12 stages:

1. Define the problem.
2. Choose those to survey.
3. Choose the type of questions.
4. Design the questionnaire.
5. Undertake a pilot survey (include data entry and analysis).
6. Make amendments and update the questionnaire.
7. Undertake the main survey.
8. Commence data entry.
9. Follow up non-responses.
10. Check the data input for errors.
11. Analyse the data.
12. Present the findings.

Selecting the sample and designing the questionnaire are two important aspects of the survey process. Time spent on these two aspects will help you undertake a worthwhile survey. You need to ask yourself who you need to target. A list of all possible candidates from which a random sample will be obtained, known as the 'sampling frame' is necessary. It is important that you only include the ones you are interested in and no others (issue of eligibility) as an inadequate sampling frame will introduce unnecessary bias (see Chapter 6).

An example of a survey questionnaire is given in Appendix A (Hughes, 2010).

Questionnaires

Questionnaires are recognised as being a very valuable data collection tool and are often used to record quantitative data. *'A questionnaire can be described as a method that seeks written or verbal responses from people to a written set of questions or statements'* (Parahoo, 2006, p. 283). In surveys, a questionnaire is frequently used to record data, however, the term questionnaire is often used to describe a survey. It is important to note that the questionnaire is a data collection tool and a survey is a research design (non-experimental). It has been reported by Brindle *et al.* (2005) that a questionnaire is the most commonly used data collection technique in midwifery. Questionnaires can have both closed and open-ended questions, and can therefore incorporate qualitative aspects in some of the questions.

The main advantages of a questionnaire is that a large sample can be sent to many locations and it is less time consuming when compared to undertaking face-to-face interviews (Holloway & Wheeler, 2002). Most questionnaires are postal, occasionally some may be telephone but using the internet is becoming a popular distribution alternative. Questionnaires can be attached and sent via email or a specific webpage questionnaire can be designed. Most universities and hospital research and development units have access to IT specialists who can help.

Questionnaires may be financially more viable than interviews, when considering that a researcher may have to travel some distance to interview participants in their own homes and the cost of their time. However, this can be influenced by the distribution method and how many questionnaires are being sent out. The cost of stationery and postage needs to be considered as well.

One thing to consider when using a questionnaire is the response rate: some people will not respond. Some people will just ignore the questionnaire and put it in the bin but some of the sample will genuinely mean to respond to you but will have not get around to it. You need to be aware of this and allow some time to send out a second reminder and questionnaire to increase the response rate. Ideally, a response rate of over 50% is regarded as a good rate; any less and the data could be viewed as not a true reflection of the views of participants (Rees, 2003; Brett-Davies, 2007). It is, therefore, essential that you seek advice and help with how to design firstly, a covering letter and secondly, a questionnaire to encourage participants to respond.

Covering letter

A covering letter needs to be user-friendly and polite; first impressions do make a difference. The letter needs to include a short introduction about the study, why it is important, anonymity and confidentiality assurances, general information about the questionnaire, i.e. estimated time to complete, how the data will be used, who you are and your address and contact details to enable participants to return the completed questionnaire. Including a stamped or franked addressed envelope will encourage more participants to respond. (For an example of a covering letter, see Appendix B.)

Designing a questionnaire

Questionnaires work best with standardised questions that are usually closed and to which structured responses are required, but some optional open-ended questions can be included to give participants an opportunity to express their personal opinions and views. Questionnaires tend to be used to gather descriptive and explanatory research that records facts and knowledge, opinions and views, behaviour and beliefs, attitudes and attributes. Generally, each participant is asked the same set of questions in a predetermined order, which Dillman (2007) describes as a *tailored design method*'. However, the task of designing a questionnaire should not be underestimated and you will need to collect precise data to answer the research question and to meet the aim and objectives of your research. It is important to remember that the design of a questionnaire will affect the response rate and the reliability and validity of the data collected. Question(s) can be adopted or adapted from other questionnaires but you will need to check for any copyright restrictions. If there are copyright restrictions you will need permission to use the material and always reference the source. Some questionnaire design software includes question type options. There are internet-based question banks, such as ESRC Question Bank which is a database of questions of UK Social Survey. For further information, see website http://survey.net.ac.uk. Nevertheless, you will have to make some compromises when designing a questionnaire as it will be unique to your research (Saunders *et al.*, 2009).

When designing a questionnaire you need to make sure you set aside enough preparation time and ask yourself what is the purpose of this questionnaire. You will have to consider what questions you want to ask and the way you want to ask them. There are no rules on how many questions you should include but remember you only need to include what is absolutely necessary as you do not want to irritate the participant and end up with a low response rate (Denscombe, 2003). The time and resources you have available will influence the design of your questionnaire and you will also need to consider:

- what type of questions to include;
- the wording of the questions;
- the order in which to ask certain questions;
- piloting the questionnaire;
- how to distribute the questionnaire;
- how the questionnaires will be returned.

Remember! Questionnaires are a good way of collecting certain types of data quickly and relatively cheaply. The majority of the data collected will be analysed by a computer software package and responses need to be coded at the questionnaire design stage.

When designing the questionnaire you also need to consider:

- informed consent;
- appearance;
- layout;
- typing;
- instructions must be clear;
- spacing between questions;
- allowing space for coding.

Types of questions

Questions can be divided into closed- and open-ended. There are six types of closed-ended questions: category, list, ranking, rating, quantity and matrix (Saunders *et al.*, 2009). The types of questions to be included in a questionnaire will depend on the research question and type of data you want to collect. Occasionally, vignettes maybe used to describe a scenario and then participants are asked how they would deal with the situation. Questions in a questionnaire need to be logical, easy to read and flow to help participants answer correctly. Filter questions and linking phrases can help. Filter questions allow participants to skip some questions that are not applicable to them, but they should be used sparingly. Sometimes a check question is included in the questionnaire to test for reliability and consistency. This involves asking a question twice but in a different way.

Open-ended questions tend to take more time to complete as the participants need to take more time to record their own personal responses in their own words. Demographic details such as age range, gender, marital status, education, occupation are usually collected in the first section of the questionnaire and are useful to confirm if the sample is representative of the general population and to investigate whether there are any correlations between personal variables.

Examples of closed-ended questions
Category
Male ☐ Female ☐ (please tick ✓ one box)

List
Which of the following midwifery pre-registration courses does your university offer?
   (please tick ✓ all boxes that apply)

☐ BSc (Hons) Midwifery – 3-year course
☐ DipHE/Advanced Diploma of Higher Education Midwifery (3-year course)
☐ BSc (Hons) Midwifery – 18-month shortened course
☐ Other

Ranking
Please number each of the factors listed below in order of importance to you that will promote a positive birth experience for a woman. Number the most important as 1, the next as 2 and so on.

☐ Kindness
☐ Safe environment
☐ Good preparation
☐ Woman in control
☐ Partner involved

Rating
Which of the following best describes your last clinical placement experience?

a) Excellent
b) Very Good

c) Good
d) Fair
e) Poor

A semantic rating scale uses a series of bipolar rating scales (pairs of opposite adjectives). For example:

Please rate how you feel about your midwifery studies

| Unmotivated | ↓---↓---↓---↓---↓---↓---↓---- | Motivated |
| Unenthusiastic | ↓---↓---↓---↓---↓---↓---↓---- | Enthusiastic |

Quantity
The response to a quantity question is always a number. For example:

If applicable, in the last 24 hours, how many cooling treatments have you applied to the area where the stitches are? □

Matrix
A matrix (grid) type of question allows you to record responses to two or more similar questions at the same time:

	A lot of the time	Some of the time	Occasionally have time	Never have time
1 Do you feel you have sufficient time to discuss the antenatal care pathway with women?				
2 Do you feel you have sufficient time to discuss how to prepare for birth?				
3 Do you feel you have sufficient time to discuss infant feeding?				

Filter question
Q10. Have you been qualified as a midwife for more than 2 years?
 Yes □ No □
 If 'no' go to question 15

Q11. Have you undertaken any continual professional development courses?
 Yes □ No □

Check question
Formula-fed babies are more likely to be overfed than breast-fed babies
Strongly disagree □ Disagree □ Neutral □ Agree □ Strongly agree □

Breast-fed babies are more likely to be overfed than formula-fed babies
Strongly disagree □ Disagree □ Neutral □ Agree □ Strongly agree □

Example of an open-ended question
Please will you give some examples of advice about diet and nutrition you would discuss with a pregnant woman
....
....
....
....
....
....

Try to avoid asking double questions, leading questions, presuming questions or hypothetical questions. For example:

• Double questions: Did you have antenatal classes at the Health Centre and the Hospital?
• Leading questions: Do you agree that smoking will affect the health of your baby?
• Presuming questions: What type of analgesia have you taken?
• Hypothetical questions: If you were having triplets would you consider having a home birth?

Other information
Clear instructions explaining how the participant returns the completed questionnaire to you need to be included at the end of the questionnaire. It is important to thank the participant for taking the time to complete the questionnaire and always include your contact details. See Appendix C.

Validity and reliability of the questionnaire
It is important to test the questionnaire design. Piloting the questionnaire should be undertaken to test the reliability of the questionnaire. In addition, **internal consistency,** which is a measure of the precision of the measuring tool (questionnaire) in a study, can be tested. One way to assess internal consistency is to use the test–retest method; this is where the same test is administered again after a time interval. However, this often proves too difficult to achieve due to time constraints.

Cronbach's alpha is a useful statistic for assessing the internal consistency of a questionnaire. It measures scores on similar items to see if there is a relationship and uses a split halves test method which means dividing a test into two halves. For example, a questionnaire to measure midwives' motivation could be divided into odd and even questions. The results from both halves are statistically analysed, and if there is weak correlation between the two this would indicate a reliability problem with the test and the questions would need to be amended.

There is also a number of validity tests that can be used to test the reliability of the questionnaire. The main ones are described as content validity, criterion-related validity and construct validity. These tests will confirm that the questionnaire is able to measure what it is supposed to be measuring.

Content validity

Content validity relates to the extent to which the questions in the questionnaire represent the phenomenon being studied. It is important that you know your topic so you can include relevant questions that need investigating and avoid irrelevant questions. For example, if a researcher wants to find out midwives' knowledge about what foods are healthy and what foods are not then sufficient sets of questions should be included to cover all aspects of diet and nutrition. Ideally, to assess content validity the designed questionnaire is reviewed by experts who can suggest how to improve on the design. There is no statistical test for content validity but the quality of the design can be measured by the level of agreement between the experts.

Criterion-related validity

Data from other related questionnaires can be used to compare the criteria to be included in your questionnaire. If the data included is similar then it can be said that the questionnaire has criterion-related validity. There are two types of criterion-related validity, concurrent and predictive (Parahoo, 2006). Concurrent relates to other current criteria with which comparisons can be made whilst predictive relates to data available in the future that will confirm if the data collected in your questionnaire is valid.

Construct validity

This type of validity relates to how well a questionnaire can measure a specific construct such as happiness, health and well-being, motivation etc. These constructs can be difficult to define and measure. A researcher will need to design questions in a questionnaire that can achieve this and demonstrate that the construct validity of the design is robust and able to measure the intended construct. Saunders *et al.* (2009, p. 373) describe construct validity as answering the question *'How well can you generalize from your measurement questions to your construct?'*

Internet resources

A good resource to create and administer questionnaires on-line is software provided by Survey Monkey available at www. surveymonkey.com. There are also other alternative software packages available such as Snap Surveys and Sphinx Development. These packages can help you design, collect, enter and analyse data. Survey Monkey offer a free service for ten or less questionnaires and when undertaking a pilot study this service maybe helpful. When undertaking the main study the costs need to be considered and this type of service may be a reasonable option. A qualitative study that explored parent's perceptions of what constitutes support for breastfeeding with a particular focus upon paternal support used the Survey Monkey resource (Tohotoa *et al.*, 2009). The reason the researchers chose this data collection option was following limited success accessing fathers via focus groups. The questions asked were the same as the ones prepared for the focus groups and telephone interviews and included open-ended questions to give fathers an opportunity to express their views.

Administering the questionnaire

Basically, there are two ways in which questionnaires are administered, those being self-administered and researcher-administered. Self-administered questionnaires are completed by the participants and it is essential to include clear written instructions on how to answer the questions. It is usually posted with a covering letter and a brief introduction included on the first page of the questionnaire to encourage people to participate and complete the questionnaire. It can, however, be delivered and collected by hand. Researcher-administered questionnaires are where the answers are recorded by the researcher on behalf of the participant. This can be undertaken in person as a face-to-face interview or by telephone. Using a computer (laptop) is also an option and responses can be recorded and entered at the same time as collecting the data. There are useful software packages such as Computer-Aided Telephone Interviewing (CATI) and Computer-Aided Personal Interviewing (CAPI) to help, and these are financially viable for large-scale research (Saunders *et al.*, 2009).

It is advised to keep a record of who has replied on a separate list, so that a reminder may be sent if no reply is received.

Data input

At the outset when you are designing the questionnaire, a coding framework needs to be developed to assist with data input for analysis of results. Data input is generally straightforward for closed-ended questions and answers can be manually entered into a database but it is important to have some sort of cross-checking system in place as errors can happen and incorrect code numbers can be entered. Where research involves a large sample, the responses can be automated. Participants' responses/answers can be read by using an optical mark reader which recognises and converts recorded answer 'marks' into data extremely quickly (Saunders *et al.*, 2009).

See Appendix A and Appendix C.

Summary

This chapter has focused on how to collect data. It has covered data collection tools and techniques that can be used to gather both qualitative and quantitative evidence. The information and guidance written in this chapter will assist midwives and students to conduct either a qualitative or quantitative research study. Knowledge and an understanding of which data collection tool and techniques fits best with a qualitative or quantitative approach are very important so this chapter has explored and covered this aspect. Researchers choose the most suitable data collection tool and techniques that will help them to answer the research question.

Data collection involves some form of observing, assessing, measuring, recording, analysing, interpreting and reporting. In midwifery, it will usually involve women, their babies and families, midwives and students, or it may relate to some policy or practice element. Midwifery research is undertaken in several settings and can be either prospective or retrospective. Data collected is related to either exploring views and experiences or testing out treatments or interventions and evaluating ways of working. This chapter has covered all these aspects to help midwives and students gain an understanding of how to collect meaningful data.

It is most likely that either a research interview or questionnaire method will be a data collection tool chosen that a midwife or student will make use of. This chapter, therefore, has given specific details on types of research interviews, how to undertake a research interview and has included examples to give midwives and students some ideas. It has also explored how to design a questionnaire and used examples of different types of questions and included some questionnaires that have been used in midwifery research.

The chapter has highlighted the importance of piloting and validating data collection tools. It is essential to evaluate and confirm the precision and effectiveness of data collection methods to gather evidence as this strengthens the quality of the research design and gives reviewers confidence in the findings. Collecting data from participants requires consideration of ethical issues and research governance. The next chapter will cover these important aspects.

CHAPTER 5

5 Ethics and research governance

Introduction

This chapter will introduce ethics and the importance of research governance. It will cover the history of how unethical research prompted the development of setting standards to govern acceptable research that addresses protectionism and the rights and dignity of participants. Ethical issues relating to midwifery research will be explored and discussed. The preparation and process of getting ethical approval for a research study will be further discussed and this will assist midwives and students to prepare a research proposal that they may then want to submit to an ethics committee. It is envisaged that midwives and students will gain some knowledge and skills to enable them to apply for ethical approval and to then confidently deal with ethical issues that may arise during the undertaking of a research study.

Aim

The aim of this chapter is to introduce midwives and students to ethics and research governance and for them to explore and understand some ethical issues relating to midwifery research. It is also intended that midwives and students will gain an insight into the preparation and process involved when designing a research proposal and gaining ethical approval.

Learning outcomes

By the end of this chapter midwives and students:

- will be aware of the importance of ethics and research governance;
- will have gained some knowledge and an understanding of ethical issues in midwifery research;
- will be able to identify ethical considerations when preparing a research proposal;
- will have gained some basic skills to prepare a research proposal to be submitted to an ethics committee;
- will have gained knowledge and skills to assist them through the process when applying for ethical approval.

The Handbook of Midwifery Research, First Edition. Mary Steen and Taniya Roberts.
© 2011 Mary Steen and Taniya Roberts. Published 2011 by Blackwell Publishing Ltd.

Introducing ethics and research

The overall aim of health research is to improve the general health and well-being of people. Clinical research with humans is justifiable as it seeks knowledge that not only is of theoretical interest but will also benefit many people and society as a whole. Health research has a wide remit but in general it is undertaken to improve the understanding of the aetiology and pathogenesis of disease, diagnostic, therapeutic, and prophylactic procedures, to develop care pathways and the impact this has upon society and the individual. It is essential that beneficial results of experiments and studies are applied to human beings to further knowledge and science to help improve the health and well-being of humanity; but health research can sometimes involve hazards and these have to be considered. How can the protection, rights and dignity of individuals be reconciled with the demands of scientific enterprise and research?

The interests of science and society should never take precedence over considerations related to the well-being of participants but, like the economy, research has become a global affair, thus raising concerns about possible exploitation of the population at large, especially disadvantaged groups. Research can be big business, some researchers may have investments and financial entanglements of all kinds with sponsors, thus prompting worries about 'conflict of interests' (Emanuel, 2002). Ethical considerations, therefore, are an integral part of a research study and researchers have an obligation to ensure that the research is ethically designed and conducted. Ethics has to take into account age, disability, gender, sexual orientation, race, culture and religion to achieve an all-inclusive approach to healthcare. The need to be transparent and declare any conflict of interests is also of the utmost importance. When planning any on-line research some additional ethical considerations may need to be considered such as privacy and confidentiality issues (Haigh & Jones, 2008). In addition, becoming a member of the Association of Internet Researchers (AoIR) may be of value; see website www.aoir.org.

History of ethics and research

Early research

In the eighteenth century, Edward Jenner tested a cowpox vaccine on his own child and other children in the neighbourhood. He found that this vaccine would protect them from smallpox (Baxby, 1981). This is an example in history that violated the rights and dignity of participants to some extent but also gave clear benefits to the general public. Unfortunately, in some cases these violations have cost participants their health or even their lives. In 1897, yellow fever was a raging epidemic and research undertaken by Guiseppe Sanarelli resulted in the isolation of the organism that caused yellow fever. To prove his claim he injected five people with the organism. His actions prompted the recognition that people were being used in experiments, possibly at great personal risk for the benefits of others, and he was heavily criticised by peers for the harm he was inflicting (McCarthy, 2001). Walter Reed was then commissioned to do further research but had to establish several 'safeguards' (Reed et al., 1901). For example, research should only involve adults and written contracts should be drawn up and signed, which included an offer of payment to the participant. Reed was also one of the first researchers to introduce the concept of the consent form. By the time of World War II, the need to obtain permission from would-be participants was widely accepted but little thought was given to the nature of this permission and to precisely what information should be disclosed to the participants.

The Nuremberg trials

In the aftermath of World War II, Nazi atrocities instigated the Nuremburg War Crime Trials (US Holocaust Memorial Museum, 2008). Twenty-three Nazi doctors and bureaucrats were tried by the Allies at Nuremburg, West Germany. Evidence that thousands of concentration camp prisoners were used in brutal experiments was reported and 1750 victims identified in the indictment were only a sample of those killed or injured; the 23 defendants were a token of these who conducted the experiments. The rationale for these experiments is impossible to understand unless one puts them within the context of Nazi Germany's overriding military aims to achieve 'racial hygiene' and in the name of 'medical research'! Narrative accounts of how different poisons were added to food and then fed to prisoners were given. The outcome was that most of these prisoners died immediately and those that did not were killed for purposes of autopsy. Freezing experiments were common and unclothed prisoners were forced to remain outdoors in freezing weather for periods of 9–14 hours or were forced to remain in a bath of freezing water for 3 hours at a time. Re-warming of the prisoners' bodies was attempted, often without success. High altitude (low pressure) experiments were undertaken on prisoners. This involved putting some prisoners into low-pressure tanks to see how long they could survive with little oxygen and some were put under water until they died and autopsies followed. Sterilisation experiments were also undertaken; prisoners were subjected to chemicals and x-rays. Horrifically, hundreds of men, women and children were killed in order to assemble a collection of skeletons for 'anthropological investigations'. It is no exaggeration to say that research ethics as a discipline 'was born in scandal and reared in protectionism' (Levine, 1996, p. 106).

Protectionism

In 1963, at the Brooklyn Jewish Disease Hospital, New York, researchers injected live cancer cells into debilitated elderly people without their fully informed consent. This lead to the hospital being sued and charges were brought against two physicians, Mandel and Southam. The two physicians claimed that the aim of the experiment was to determine the rate of rejection of cancer cells as all the evidence suggested these injected cells would cause an immune reaction and lead to their expulsion. In their medical opinion, this experiment did not present any risks and informing patients of the details would cause them needless psychological distress and therefore this minimised the risks to them.

What do you think?

The verdict was that the State of New York found it could not justify *'non-disclosure'* on a researcher–participant relationship and Mandel's and Southam's licences were suspended for 1 year (Langer, 1966).

Tuskegee Syphilis Study

A famous unethical study that violated the rights and dignity of human beings was the Tuskegee Syphilis Study (Olansky *et al.*, 1956; Corbie-Smith, 1999). This study commenced in 1932 in Macon County, Alabama. The aim of this study was to assess the natural course of syphilis which had reached epidemic proportions in African-American males in that area. However, it appears that there was no scientific rationale for the study and there was evidence from another study in Oslo at the turn of the nineteenth century that resulted in treatment of latent syphilis as standard care. The study recruited 400 African-American men who were mostly illiterate and these men were not informed about the true nature of study or about their condition; nor were their partners informed of their risk. When 'penicillin' became publicly available in the late 1940s these men were not given the opportunity to use it. In fact, efforts were made to ensure that these men did not receive treatment or become aware of it. It was not until 1972 that press reports prompted the US Secretary of the Department of Health, Education & Welfare to stop the study. By this time only 74 of the men were still alive and there was some evidence that at least 28 but perhaps more than a 100 had died directly from advanced syphilitic lesions. It was argued that this study *'exemplified a pattern of institutional racism in health care'*. In the late 1970s compensation was authorised to survivors and to families of those who died but it was not until 1997 that a formal apology was given by the US government.

A landmark article

In 1966, Henry Knowles-Beecher published the article entitled 'Ethics & Clinical Research' (Knowles-Beecher, 1966) In this article he described 22 studies that he claimed violated the basic standards of ethical research with humans, some examples were:

- a study where penicillin was withheld from soldiers with a streptococcal throat infection, even though it was known that there was a risk of developing rheumatic fever and even death from valvular disease;
- a study that involved inserting a needle into the left atrium of the heart during bronchoscopy with unknown risk and no benefits to the patient.

This landmark article raised awareness and greater demands for accountability of medical research (Kopp, 1999).

Defending medical research

In 1971, Louis Lasagna posed the rhetorical question, *'How many of medicines greatest advances might have been delayed or prevented by the rigid application of some currently proposed principles to research at large?'* (Lasagna, 1971). However, the risks versus benefits must be balanced and clear guidance to ethical and acceptable research is essential to protect and prevent the rights and dignity of participants from being violated as they have been in the past.

The Nuremberg Code

A set of standards to judge the doctors and scientists who had conducted medical experiments on prisoners of war was developed. This led to the creation of the Nuremberg Code in 1949. The Nuremburg Code is the most widely known document on ethics and research is includes ten points of *'acceptable'* research involving humans (Box 5.1).

Box 5.1 The Nuremberg Code (1949) – The International Principles.

1. The voluntary consent of the human subject is absolutely essential. This means that the person involved should have legal capacity to give consent; should be so situated as to be able to exercise free power of choice, without the intervention of any element of force, fraud, deceit, duress, over-reaching, or other ulterior form of constraint or coercion; and should have sufficient knowledge and comprehension of the elements of the subject matter involved as to enable him to make an understanding and enlightened decision. This latter element requires that before the acceptance of an affirmative decision by the experimental subject there should be made known to him the nature, duration, and purpose of the experiment; the method and means by which it is to be conducted; all inconveniences and hazards reasonably to be expected; and the effects upon his health or person which may possibly come from his participation in the experiment. The duty and responsibility for ascertaining the quality of the consent rests upon each individual who initiates, directs or engages in the experiment. It is a personal duty and responsibility which may not be delegated to another with impunity.
2. The experiment should be such as to yield fruitful results for the good of society, unprocurable by other methods or means of study, and not random and unnecessary in nature.
3. The experiment should be so designed and based on the results of animal experimentation and a knowledge of the natural history of the disease or other problem under study that the anticipated results will justify the performance of the experiment.
4. The experiment should be so conducted as to avoid all unnecessary physical and mental suffering and injury.
5. No experiment should be conducted where there is an a priori reason to believe that death or disabling injury will occur; except, perhaps, in

those experiments where the experimental physicians also serve as subjects.

6. The degree of risk to be taken should never exceed that determined by the humanitarian importance of the problem to be solved by the experiment.

7. Proper preparations should be made and adequate facilities provided to protect the experimental subject against even remote possibilities of injury, disability, or death.

8. The experiment should be conducted only by scientifically qualified persons. The highest degree of skill and care should be required through all stages of the experiment of those who conduct or engage in the experiment.

9. During the course of the experiment the human subject should be at liberty to bring the experiment to an end if he has reached the physical or mental state where continuation of the experiment seems to him to be impossible.

10. During the course of the experiment the scientist in charge must be prepared to terminate the experiment at any stage, if he has probable cause to believe, in the exercise of the good faith, superior skill and careful judgement required of him that a continuation of the experiment is likely to result in injury, disability, or death to the experimental subject.

Declaration of Helsinki

The World Medical Association developed the Declaration of Helsinki as a statement of ethical principles to provide guidance and recommendations for research involving human beings. This declaration was first introduced in 1964 and has been amended in 1975, 1983, 1989, 1996, 2000 and 2008 (World Medical Association, 2008). The current version should be used and the previous versions should only be cited for historical purposes. For further information see website http://www.wma.net/en/30publications/10policies/b3/index.html.

These landmark documents have set international regulations and ethics standards to protect the public when being involved in research. These standards are to assure that research involving humans is carried out in an ethical manner.

Principles of ethics

Ethical guidelines and principles have been developed to protect and safeguard people's rights and dignity. Ethical approval strengthens the credibility of a qualitative study or validity of a quantitative study and safeguards participants' interests.

Four basic principles that underpin ethics and are relevant to research that involves human beings are:

- respect for autonomy;
- non-maleficence;
- beneficience;
- justice.

To gain ethical approval a researcher will have to demonstrate that participants have autonomy and that their wishes are respected, harm will be avoided, any benefits will outweigh the risks and they will be treated fairly (Beauchamp & Childress, 2001; Riddick-Thomas, 2009).

It is helpful to consider the use of a standardised ethical considerations criterion to assess the feasibility of undertaking a study. It is important that you provide an ethics committee with sufficient evidence that the research study you are proposing has considered the four main ethical principles mentioned above. In addition, the four principles listed below will help you understand what has to be made crystal clear to an ethics committee before approval will be granted when undertaking midwifery research:

- respect for the women;
- the duty to do good for the women;
- the duty not to do harm to the women;
- demonstrable fairness.

Remember, it is vitally important that as researchers you need to be knowledgeable about the ethical issues that need to be considered when planning a research study. To guard participants from harm, the following six ethical principles are described by Parahoo (2006, p. 112):

- **beneficence** – the research project should benefit the participating individual and society in general;
- **non-maleficence** – the research should not cause any harm to participants (physical/psychological);
- **fidelity** – there should be trust between researchers and participants;
- **justice** – the researchers should be fair to the participants;
- **veracity** – the researcher must tell the truth;
- **confidentiality** – must be respected.

Informed consent is a vital part of conducting an ethically designed research study. Autonomy is considered to be the seventh ethical research principle (McHaffie, 2000), whereby the potential research participants have the right to decide whether to take part in the research or not. Therefore, the researcher has a moral obligation to ensure that the participants are fully informed of the following (Lindsay, 2007; Haigh, 2008):

- full disclosure of the details of the study;
- the identification of the researcher and organisation;

- the nature of the participation;
- informed that they need not volunteer;
- assured they have the right to withdraw at any time without any negative consequences;
- assurance of confidentiality;
- assurance of anonymity;
- be given the opportunity to ask questions;
- absence of pressure/coercion;
- time is taken by the researcher to ensure that the information being given is understood;
- consent should be given both verbally and in writing.

A major ethical consideration for a midwife conducting research is to be aware that a pregnant woman is considered to be vulnerable and particular thought is required when planning the research design to take this into account. The vulnerability relates to the pregnant woman being responsible, not just for her life, but for that of her fetus and subsequent newborn. For example *'you must show that your recruitment procedure does not put any pressure on the women related to their pregnancy'* (Shields & Winch, 2008, p. 35). It would be deemed unacceptable to approach and recruit women whilst they are in labour. Therefore recruitment and consent should take place in the antenatal period if the study is to take place whilst a woman is in labour and should be re-confirmed before the researcher enters the delivery room, to ensure that coercion is not applied. Likewise approaching a woman immediately post-delivery is also undesirable. Therefore careful thought has to be put into recruitment of your sample (participants).

In experimental research, the sample size has the potential to be of ethical concern as there are the statistical issues to consider – a power calculation is vital to determine the amount of participants needed. Too few make it impossible to determine/test the hypothesis and too many may not be required.

As to data collection, during an interview questions should be carefully selected and asked in a sensitive manner (phenomenology). When observation is undertaken it is deemed unethical not to inform people that they are being observed (ethnography) (Davies, 2007). In experimental research, particularly a randomised controlled trial, the group that are either to receive no treatment or the placebo, must consider this option to be acceptable (Smith, 2008), as the overarching issue in any conducted research is firstly to cause no harm.

Pseudonyms must be used to maintain confidentiality and any collected data must be carefully stored in a locked cabinet. It must be stressed that identifying information about the participants must be stored separately to the data that will be utilised in the study, and that this material should not identify who the participants are. How long this information is stored is dependent on whether the organisation involved with the research has the ability to store secure archive material (Griffiths, 2009).

Another consideration is the organisation of psychological support following participation in a research study, which may have the potential of unintentionally causing memories or events to be relived, which may be distressing. When planning the study *Women's experiences of obstetric emergencies* (Mapp & Hudson, 2005), it was vital that this concern was realised. As part of the consent process the participants were asked if their GPs could be informed of their participation in the research study and this was agreed by all. The services of a psychologist were provided and offered to all participants, once data collection (interviews) had taken place.

Once the study is completed the ethical researcher should give feedback to participants. In a large randomised controlled trial this may not always be possible, although it should be possible in a qualitative study; if it is not then some indication of where and when the results will be disseminated should be provided. With regards to dissemination, the researcher has an obligation to the participants to report and disseminate the results, and on publication of the findings any bias or limitations should be reported (Rees, 2003).

In summary ethical considerations are an integral component to planning and conducting research. If you as the researcher have not considered them, then your suitability to conduct research will be in question. Whatever the context, the interests of participants come first and researcher(s) must be satisfied that they have taken all reasonable steps to protect the dignity, rights, safety and well-being of participants.

Research governance

Research governance defines the principles for undertaking and disseminating good quality research. It is essential to ensure that research is conducted to a very high standard and that ethical issues have been considered and addressed prior to and for the duration of the study. Research governance is one of the core standards for healthcare organisations and applies to a full range of research approaches and methods.

As a general rule research should meet the same standards of governance that adhere to internationally recognised standards of good practice. However, there are elements of risk with regard to the terms of return on investment and the safety and well-being of participants. Any risks, pain or discomfort to participants must be kept to a minimum. Balancing the proportionate risks with the guidance for good practice needs to be agreed. Risks have to be transparent and managed appropriately. Researchers must demonstrate that they have taken all necessary steps to protect participants' rights, dignity, safety, health and well-being. Research governance aims to limit poor practice, adverse incidents, misconduct and fraud. It plays a role in ensuring that lessons are learned and shared when poor practice is identified.

Research governance provides a structure for new ideas and innovation which can then be effectively transferred as knowledge, new technologies and tools, skills and training, and ultimately promote best practice to improve the

Box 5.2 Research governance – principles, requirements and standards.

- Defines mechanisms to deliver.
- Describes monitoring and assessment arrangements.
- Improves research and safeguards the public by:
  - enhancing ethical awareness and scientific quality
  - promoting good practice
  - reducing adverse incidents and ensuring lessons are learned
  - forestalling poor performance and misconduct.
- Is for all those who:
  - design research studies
  - participate in research
  - host research in their organisations
  - fund research proposals or infrastructure
  - manage research
  - undertake research.
- Is for managers and staff in all professional groups, no matter how senior or junior.
- Is for those working in all health and social care environments including:
  - primary care
  - secondary care
  - tertiary care
  - social care
  - public health.

quality of services and care. Achieving high-quality research, however, depends heavily upon good cooperation between all those involved.

The Department of Health has published and recently modified the second edition of a document entitled *Research Governance Framework for Health & Social Care* (Department of Health, 2005). This document outlines the principles of **good governance** that apply to research undertaken within the NHS and Social Care services. This document clearly sets out principles, requirements and standards of research governance in a helpful bullet point format. See Box 5.2.

The Department of Health Research Governance Framework also covers research undertaken using resources of health and social care organisations and any research involving industry, charities, research councils and universities within health and social care systems that can have an impact on the quality of services.

In the UK, each of the four countries has a Research Governance Framework for Health and Social Care and similar frameworks are in place in other countries. It is important to gain the general public's confidence in midwifery research. It is, therefore, essential that maternity care services have systems in place to ensure the principles and requirements of research governance are consistently applied to research, which can include both clinical and non-clinical studies. Good governance is a key component for high-quality research. Women, their babies and families have a right to expect a high standard of research that is ethically sound and transparent.

Ethical issues relating to midwifery research

The midwifery research community have a responsibility to work towards being better informed about ethical issues and up-to-date knowledge of the relevant legal and governance regulations.

Informed consent

When involving people (general public and staff) or information relating to them in research, it is a legal requirement to obtain ethical approval before you commence recruiting and collecting data. A researcher must demonstrate evidence in the proposal that gaining informed consent has been addressed (NMC, 2008).

Informed consent is absolutely necessary to protect and safeguard people but there is some controversy that exists over the nature and possibility of a person giving their informed consent. However, there is some agreement that the consent process can be assessed by how the information, comprehension and voluntariness for participants are considered (Belmont Report, 1979). For further information access the Office of Human Subjects Research website and search Regulations and Ethical Guidelines; see website http://ohsr.od.nih.gov/guidelines/belmont.html#go1. For an example of a standardised consent form see Figure 5.1.

Research protocol and information sheet

A clear and concise explanation of how you plan to undertake the research is given by designing a proposal that includes a research protocol and user-friendly information sheet. These two elements will be required by ethics committees. An ethics committee will need to consider the proposed process of obtaining individual consent from each participant or their parent/guardian if under 18 years of age (there are usually a specific ethics committee for research involving minors) is going to be achieved. It is a requirement that within the research proposal there is a specific section that gives details on how the research governance aspects of the study are to be met. These include: the transparency of information to be given and collected during the undertaking of the study; obtaining verbal and written consent; the collection of personal details; anonymity and confidentiality assurance; secure storage of data collected, in particular any personal information gathered; and how these elements will be monitored and managed. In addition, it is usual to note that ethics committees require evidence of a plan on how you will disseminate

Title of project:

Name of researcher:

Please initial box

1. I confirm that I have read and understood the
participant information sheet, dated ....,
for the above study and have had the opportunity
to ask questions.

2. I understand that my participation is voluntary
and that I am free to withdraw at any time, without
giving any reason and without my care or legal rights
being affected.

3. I understand that sections of any of my maternity notes
may be looked at by responsible individuals from
regulatory authorities where it is relevant to my taking
part in research. I give permission for these individuals
to have access to my records.

4. I agree to take part in the above study.

_____   _____   _____
Name of participant   Date   Signature

_____   _____   _____
Name of person taking consent Date   Signature
(if different from researcher)

_____   _____   _____
Researcher   Date   Signature

Figure 5.1 Example consent form.

your findings. A copy of a written report should be made available to all participants, the ethics committee, funding bodies, the study hospital and associated academic institution. A commitment to write a publication and give a conference paper on the study findings within a specified timeframe should be included as a goal.

A 12-point guide for designing a participant information sheet:

1. Commence with what the research study is about, who is responsible for undertaking the study and
2. Include information about how long the study is expected to take.
3. Invite them to participate and explain why you have asked them to participate in the study.
4. Explain what they will have to do if they consent to participate.
5. Explain where the study will take place and how privacy will ensured.
6. Explain how the information will be collected, for example, a short questionnaire, being interviewed and recorded via an audio-tape and on how many occasions.
7. Explain that there will be an opportunity to discuss their responses to ensure that you have understood correctly what they have recorded or said.
8. Discuss who will have access to the information and how the information will be analysed and stored.
9. Explain how the information will be shared with relevant health professionals and the public, e.g. a written report, a publication, a presentation.
10. Explain that their involvement in the study will remain confidential and their identity will not be disclosed. Give details of any coding system to be used to ensure anonymity.
11. Explain that participation is totally voluntary and they do not have to take part if they are not happy to do so or can withdraw at any time if they change their mind.
12. Finally, give details of who to contact if they have any concerns or would like to discuss the study further.

An example of an information leaflet is given in Appendix D.

Gaining ethical approval

You can obtain guidance on gaining ethical approval from your place of work or academic institution. Both organisations have ethics committees and if you are undertaking a postgraduate qualification that involves undertaking a research study you will need approval from both. In addition, you will need to register your research study and gain approval from your local hospitals' research and development units, to ensure research governance requirements have been met. If you are going to undertake research in the UK which involves the NHS in some way, for example pregnant women accessing maternity services or health professionals, then you will need to access Integrated Research Access System (IRAS) online at www.myproject.org.uk.

Integrated Research Access System (IRAS)

IRAS is a collaborative initiative supported by several organisations which provides a single, integrated on-line application system. It was set up in January 2008 to streamline the ethical approval process to conduct health and social care research. Using IRAS, researchers can enter information about their study in one place. It is designed to save time and effort and a researcher only has to complete one application form. The system has helpful prompts and an e-learning module to guide you. This may be a challenging task if you have never applied for ethical approval before. Many midwives and students have found the length of the on-line application form initially off-putting but, with perseverance and patience, have successfully completed the form. IRAS do take into consideration users' views and are continually taking steps to improve the on-line process. So, if you do have any suggestions or comments when completing an on-line application which you feel may improve the service, please do not hesitate to contact the IRAS team. For further information see https://www.myresearchproject.org.uk/Help/Updates.aspx.

Research passport

If you are a midwife who does not have a contractual agreement with the NHS, e.g. working in higher education or a private birth centre, and are proposing to undertake research which involves NHS patients, facilities or data then you will need to obtain what is known as a research passport.

To safeguard vulnerable groups the National Institute for Health Research (NIHR) has developed a research passport system. This system has been devised to meet the standards for employment checks required in the NHS which has been adapted to meet the requirements of a recently introduced vetting and barring scheme (VBS). Once the checks have been validated a letter of access or honorary research contract is then issued by the host NHS organisation and permission to undertake the research is granted. This permission can be for a specific research study or for a period of 3 years. For further information, *A Good Practice Resource Pack* can be downloaded at http://www.nihr.ac.uk/systems/Pages/systems_research_passports.aspx.

Ethics committees

Ethics committees are convened to provide independent advice to participants, researchers, funders, sponsors, employers, healthcare services and health professionals that research studies will be undertaken ethically. Ethics committees are one of a series of **safeguards**. Fundamentally, ethics committees' role and responsibilities are to:

- provide independent advice on the extent to which proposals for research studies to be carried out within a health service comply with recognised ethical standards;
- conduct a robust review to ensure that the research study has considered ethical issues and adheres to ethical principles;

- protect the rights, safety, dignity and well-being of all actual and potential participants;
- protect primarily individuals who will be participating in research but also researchers and health professionals.

Any concerns or clarifications will need to be addressed before ethical approval will be granted. (Department of Health, 2001, 2005) A checklist of questions to help midwives consider ethical issues when undertaking midwifery research has been adapted from RCM Masterclasses for Research (2006). See Box 5.3.

Society has a duty of care to ensure that research governance, ethical review regulatory processes and good quality standards are in place to protect the rights, dignity and safety of all research participants.

Box 5.3 Ethical issues and midwifery research.

The research study
- Has the researcher undertaken some research education and training and do they have the experience to undertake the research?
- Has adequate supervision and support to undertake the research study been organised?
- Is the research needed?
- Has the researcher demonstrated evidence to justify the need?
- Is the research question answerable?
- Is there evidence of a well designed research proposal?
- Has the proposal been peer-reviewed (minimum two reviewers)?
- Is the research relevant to midwifery practice?
- Are the most appropriate methods going to be used?
- Have the research tools and techniques been tested?
- How reliable will the research findings be?
- How will the evidence be disseminated?

Ethical issues
- Has the researcher(s) considered the risks versus benefits when carrying out the proposed study?
- Have health and safety aspects for both participants, researcher and staff been considered?
- Has ethical approval been applied for? (if applicable – application completed on-line)
- Has the research been ethically reviewed by an ethics committee?
- Have service-users been involved in the design of the study?
- How will service-users be involved in the undertaking of the study?
- Have their rights, dignity and safety been considered?
- Do any participants come from disadvantaged groups?

- If so, have their rights, dignity and safety been considered further to protect them from unnecessary harm?
- How will confidentiality be ensured?
- How will participants remain anonymous throughout the research?
- How will their consent be obtained (verbal and written)?
- Has adequate time been given to ask questions?
- Has the opportunity for further explanation and questions been considered?
- Will there be clear details on how to contact the researcher?
- How will potential participants be made aware that they are free to withdraw at any time during the research?
- In addition, will it be made very clear to participants who withdraw that this will not affect their treatment or care in anyway?

Funding issues
- How is the research study to be funded?
- Has a cost evaluation been undertaken?
- Is there any commercial funding supporting the research?
- Are participants to be reimbursed for their time, travel costs, expenses?
- Will any tokens of gratitude (such as book tokens, vouchers) be offered as a recognition of valuing the participants' time and efforts?
- Will any incentives (financial or otherwise) be offered to participants?

Summary

This chapter has introduced the role of ethics when undertaking research and has discussed the importance of research governance. Overall, health research is undertaken to improve the general health and well-being of people. However, it is vitally important that research is undertaken ethically and safely. The history of how unethical research prompted the development of setting standards to govern acceptable research that addresses protectionism and the rights and dignity of participants has been covered. An insight into the historical perspective of healthcare ethics is essential for midwives and students to gain an understanding of why it is important to obtain ethical approval for their research studies.

It is also important that midwives and students learn how to manage and monitor their research activities to ensure that research is undertaken to the best of their ability. The principles of research governance and where to find useful information have been included to help midwives and students to gain knowledge and understanding.

It is envisaged that after reading and working through this chapter, midwives and students will have gained knowledge and skills about how to apply for ethical approval and to then confidently deal with ethical issues that may arise during the undertaking of a research study. In addition, midwives and students will have gained some insight into how to prepare, manage and monitor a research study.

It is important to be honest and transparent when analysing data and the next chapter focuses on data analysis.

6 Data analysis

Introduction to data analysis

How do you make sense of the data? This chapter will introduce midwives and students to the basic principles of data analysis. Some qualitative and quantitative data analysis methods will be explored and discussed. Examples of data analysis of midwifery research undertaken by the authors and others will be used to demonstrate and clarify some qualitative and quantitative data analysis methods. A basic understanding of descriptive and inferential statistics will be discussed to reduce some of the anxieties midwives and students have when undertaking research. It is envisaged that midwives and students will have increased confidence and competencies to analyse both qualitative and quantitative data and then use this new knowledge to guide their clinical practice.

Aims

The aims of this chapter are:

- to introduce midwives and students to the principles of data analysis;
- to explore both qualitative and quantitative data analysis methods;
- to give midwives and students an insight into the advantages and disadvantages of both qualitative and quantitative data analysis methods and some basic knowledge of the use of statistics.

Learning outcomes

By the end of this chapter midwives and students:

- will have gained knowledge and an understanding of the principles of data analysis;
- will have gained some knowledge and an understanding of qualitative data analysis methods;
- will have gained some knowledge and an understanding of quantitative data analysis methods;
- will be able to identify the differences between qualitative and quantitative data analysis methods;
- will be able to use their knowledge to assist them to undertake both qualitative and quantitative data analysis.

The Handbook of Midwifery Research, First Edition. Mary Steen and Taniya Roberts.
© 2011 Mary Steen and Taniya Roberts. Published 2011 by Blackwell Publishing Ltd.

Qualitative data analysis

Introduction

Some type of manual analysis of the data will need to be undertaken by reading and re-reading the transcripts, making marginal notes, identifying key words and phrases, sub-themes, main themes and a core theme, and the data can generate further ideas for further research. This hands-on approach can be time consuming and so it is acceptable to employ others to assist with the analysis and this has the advantage of reducing researcher bias. Ideally, another researcher or your supervisor should independently analyse the data as well as yourself and then collectively you should compare and contrast your interpretative findings and come to some agreement about the meaning of the data.

The main concept behind qualitative data is to produce major themes; quotes can support this (Brett-Davies, 2007). There are several qualitative data analysis frameworks to guide a researcher when undertaking a thematic analysis. There are also specifically designed computer software packages, such as NVivo, NUD*IST, ATLAS, OpenCode and QSR International, to help a researcher analyse a large amount of written data. However, as a researcher you will need to develop some IT skills to use these packages and become familiar with the applications.

One of the most important steps in the research process is the analysis of the collected data. Qualitative data analysis is a creative but time-consuming process that needs to be systematic and transparent. It has to be logical in the process, yet be open to understanding meanings from the views of the participants taking part in the research. It is subjective, yet it is easier to guard against bias if more researchers are involved in the steps in analysing the data. Qualitative data analysis can be an iterative process, whereby researchers repeatedly return to the data and reflect on their findings (Carter, 2004).

Data analysis methods

The intention of this section is to try and simplify what can sometimes be the complex analytical process of qualitative data analysis. It must however be realised that it is a creative, conceptual process, whereby meaning and interpretation are given to the data collected. There is generally one type of analysis used for qualitative research: thematic analysis. However, certain research methodologies do utilise specific data analysis frameworks. This section will explain the process of thematic analysis and outline the more specific frameworks and also consider the activity of reflexivity by the researcher.

Once the qualitative data has been collected (from interviews, observations, focus groups) it is usually transcribed into a written script. Once collected the data may be managed manually or by computer software packages, such as NVivo (Gibbs, 2002). However, the novice researcher does need to be familiar with data analysis techniques (Barbour, 2008) to enable an informed decision on how to manage the data and how to proceed with the analysis. As with

Box 6.1 Tips for managing and handling 'raw' data.

- Reference all data material with a number to correlate with when and where collected.
- Make copies of all collected data.
- Ensure all transcribed data is printed on A4 sheets.
- Ensure there is space in the margins to make notes.

Box 6.2 Stages of qualitative analysis (thematic analysis).

- Read the scripts one at a time.
- Re-read as many times as required to enable coding of the data.
- Code the data. This involves:
  - breaking down the data into units for analysis. Units may be specific words or ideas or events;
  - categorising the units, also known as open coding, '*to discover, name and categorise phenomena*' (Denscombe 2003, p. 271). This is a continual process, whereby initial categories may be changed or refined.
- Develop themes. Themes are realised from the categories.

many aspects of the research process this does require good time management and organisational skills, whether this is to meet a funding or academic deadline. This process should not be rushed; it is an interpretative journey, where meanings and understandings are reached.

Denscombe (2003, p. 270) gives recommendations for managing and handling 'raw' data (see Box 6.1). This follows the manual procedures for initially handling the data.

It is then the researcher's responsibility to analyse the collected information and to convey meaning to the transcribed text. It is a systematic process, but one that may need to be revisited many times. Box 6.2 illustrates the key stages. Whether the stages are conducted manually (a space, table, scissors, glue and lots of patience are required to cut and paste the categories under themes on a poster-sized paper) or by using a computer software package to manage the data, the process is laborious.

An example of this process is given in Box 6.3 where an extract from a transcribed interview has been categorised.

The bold print in Box 6.3 indicates an initial acknowledgement in attempting to categorise a transcript, this process will be repeated and the categories will be refined. This preliminary analysis revealed the following categories: communication; communication with colleagues; types of communication; and preferred communication. Emerging themes therefore would develop from the same categories being present in other transcripts. Once no new themes are discovered, saturation is reached. The themes are collated and a

Box 6.3 Extract of interview – experience of work environment.

> I would say that I've experienced many **different ways** of **communicating with colleagues**, from a purely **professional perspective** to engaging in **friendly conversations to being 'cold shouldered'**. I obviously **prefer the first two options**. I think that you can communicate in a **professional way and still engage in common courtesies** of acknowledging and responding when someone says 'good morning'. As to how we communicate, the **majority of sharing information is at meetings** and these are usually followed up by emailed minutes of meetings. Very rarely do I communicate by phone it's **mostly email**.

rich description or interpretation of what the events/circumstances/experiences mean to the participants is revealed and the findings of the research are uncovered.

Other examples of data analysis frameworks follow with a specific focus on phenomenology, ethnography and grounded theory research methods.

Phenomenology and data analysis

Phenomenological data analysis is usually determined by the type of phenomenology used and follows the most appropriate steps in data analysis, which is advocated by the approach. There are three main methods of analysis used in a Husserlian phenomenological approach. These are the methods devised by Colaizzi (1978), Giorgi (1985) and Van Kaam (1966) (Beck, 1994; Crotty 1996; Carpenter, 1999; Robinson, 2006). The three data analysis methods of Van Kaam, Colaizzi and Giorgi share common features, in that they all transcribe the data and this is then coded into themes. Key words are noticed in the transcripts, which then identify the themes (Robinson, 2006). There are notable differences between these methods, however. Giorgi's method, for instance, differs from Colaizzi's in that the former synthesises the grouped statements. Van Kaam's method differs from both the Colaizzi and Giorgi methods in that a hypothetical identification of the phenomenon is formulated and then tested against random chosen samples before being revised following testing on other cases and the description is finally identified (Crotty, 1996). Colaizzi's method differs from that of both Giorgi and Van Kaam, in that final validation of the study is provided by the participants who are given the description of the experience to verify. This all suggests that data analysis using a phenomenological approach is complicated (Mapp, 2008). Robinson (2006) believes, however, that Colaizzi's data analysis method is relatively user-friendly and can be used by novice or experienced researchers alike to provide a clear description of the phenomenon.

There are specific frameworks recommended for Heidegerrian (hermeneutic) phenomenological data analysis; an example is Diekelmann, Allen and

Tanner's seven-stage framework (1989, cited by Polit & Beck 2008, p. 251). Another example is described in the book *Hermeutic Phenomenological Research: a Practical Guide for Nurse Researchers* (Cohen *et al.*, 2000), which suggests that analysis should begin during the interview where the researcher should actively listen to try to establish some meaning to what is being said by the research informant. The next stage is to read the transcribed data several times, with the aim of realising an initial interpretation; coding and reduction of the data (editing what is relevant to the study or not) and then thematic analysis should follow. This should ultimately result in the researcher(s) producing a narrative interpretation of what the research participants have expressed. The authors also recommend that a research team should analyse the data, as one person would become overwhelmed with the magnitude of data that can be produced with this type of study.

Ethnography and data analysis
Ethnographic data analysis can follow the process of thematic analysis, whereby field notes and interviews are transcribed and analysed together for possible themes and meanings, allowing the observations to be more clearly understood (Price & Johnson, 2006).

Donovan (2006, p. 184) believes that *'descriptive analysis'* is the more traditional approach to use in analysing ethnographic studies; this entails the ethnographer developing *'ideas that are tested against observations and vice versa. There is a back and forth process of data collection and analysis, which involves switching from emic to etic perspectives and testing them against each other'*. This suggests that there are different approaches that can be used to analyse data collected during an ethnographic study and that analysis and interpretation can proceed in parallel (Holloway & Todres, 2006).

Grounded theory and data analysis
Grounded theory and data analysis is different to other research methods in that data collection and analysis are linked from the beginning of the research, proceed in parallel and interact continuously (Strauss & Corbin, 1998). Therefore the processes of data collection and data analysis occur in tandem and are sometimes referred to as the grounded theory approach (Rees, 2003).

Data analysis of the transcribed data is a structured process if the following principles are applied. The transcribed interviews should be read line by line and the researcher should be asking questions of the data such as 'What is this data a study of?' 'What is actually happening here?' The purpose of this is to develop *'substantive codes'*, where abstract information from the interviews is coded and then the coded or annotated material is scrutinised for patterns and or categories (Glaser, 1998). The *'constant comparative method'* is a technique peculiar to grounded theory (Bazanger, 1997), and is representative of both Glaser and Strauss's conceptual framework for this research methodology. The emerging codes and categories are constantly checked against the data that have been analysed, allowing the researcher to interpret and analyse the information and develop a theory closely linked to, i.e. *'grounded'* in, the data (Denscombe, 2003, p. 120). *'Theoretical sensitivity, whereby researchers must have the ability to immerse themselves in the data and give meaning to it'* (Bluff, 2006, p. 124), is an essential requirement of this process and is integral to grounded theory (Roberts, 2008).

Historical research and analysis
There are different methods of inquiry used to interpret textual data, depending on its source. Discourse analysis, according to Rugg and Petrie (2007, p. 159), is about *'who says what, about what, to whom, in what format'*. To them discourse analysis involves plots, narratives and conversations. It is a way of *'constructing social reality'*, a way of looking for hidden meanings within the discourse (Parahoo, 2006, p. 210).

Textual analysis could be used for newspaper stories/commentaries:

> Textual analysis is a way for researchers to gather information about how other human beings make sense of the world ... and whereby we attempt to understand the likely interpretations of texts made by people who consume them.
>
> McKee, 2003, p. 1–2

Reflexivity
To ensure the trustworthiness of the study, Kingdon (2005) recommends that researchers should engage in reflexivity, which entails adopting a self-awareness as to the potential biases that they may bring to a research study, in terms of influencing data analysis. However, to reduce bias and also to ensure rigour, more than one researcher should be involved in the process of data analysis. To further ensure trustworthiness of the research findings, the researchers must be able to illustrate their steps in the data analysis process, and demonstrate that the findings are not based on personal opinion, but on a rigorous, analytical, transparent process (Roberts, 2009).

Data-analysis and meta-synthesis
A meta-synthesis involves an analytical process similar to that undertaken when analysing an individual qualitative study. Comparisons and contrasts of metaphors, phrases, ideas, concepts, relations and themes in the original texts are analysed to establish how far the themes arising from the included studies are similar, or different; and new collective emerging themes are then developed during the analytical stages. To increase credibility and reduce researcher bias, the analysis is undertaken separately by a least two researchers and then the final analysis is agreed by consensus. In addition, reflexivity is accounted for by researchers acknowledging their own values and beliefs and then consciously seeking them as disconfirming data when undertaking the analysis. The final stage in the analytical process is the generation of a synthesis derived from the emerging themes of included studies (Noblit & Hare, 1988; Walsh & Downe, 2005).

Conclusion

Qualitative data analysis can assume different frameworks depending on the type of research involved. It is a creative process that is required to be systematic and rigorous, with researchers practising reflexivity and ensuring that their steps in the analytical process are clear and transparent.

Quantitative data analysis methods

Introduction

Quantitative data analysis has gained scientific respectability as it uses mathematical and statistical tests to measure quantifiable outcomes. It conveys a sense of solid objective research analysis. The advent of the personal computer and powerful statistical software packages have assisted in the analysis of large volumes of number-based data (number crunching) and relative novices can undertake fairly complex statistical tests (Denscombe, 2003). However, be careful as there is a risk that you could be using the wrong statistical test if you do not have sufficient knowledge of the different types of data that can be quantitatively analysed and a basic understanding of statistics! It is vital that you take time to read and study literature that will help you understand the processes and methods that are used to undertake quantitative data analysis. This will help you when preparing your research proposal as you will need to discuss what method(s) of data collection you are proposing to use and what type of analysis you will undertake. For those of you about to embark on a research study that uses a quantitative research approach where some numerical data collection and analysis are required, it is always advisable to seek advice and assistance from a statistician at the outset to guide you as to what statistical tests are suitable for the type of data you are collecting and to assist you in working out a sample size based on a power calculation estimate if this is needed.

Study validity

Internal validity

Internal validity relates to the extent to which the design and conduct of the study eliminate the possibility of bias and the results can be attributed to the treatment/intervention; in other words that the conclusions drawn about causal effects of the dependent variable on the independent variable are valid and not due to flaws in the design and conduct of the study.

External validity

External validity is the extent to which the results of a study are relevant to the population at large; in other words, the extent to which the conclusions drawn from a study can be generalised and used to represent the general public. It is another term for generalisibility.

Independent and dependent variables

The independent variable (cause in a study) is used to predict or manipulate the effect on other dependent variable(s). A dependent variable (effect in a study) depends on another variable.

For example: in a study to see if there is a relationship between student midwives' reading activity and their average grades, the reading activity would be the presumed cause (independent variable) and the grades would be the effect (dependent variable).

Cause and effect

Statistical analysis and significance involves seeking and finding out causes and associations with the data collected. Participants' characteristics and the role that chance plays can influence the findings and these aspects have to be controlled for.

What is quantitative data analysis?

Quantitative data analysis is the analysis of data which are measurable or quantifiable, such as gender or age, a baby's temperature, birth weight, or a blood pressure reading. Generally, quantitative data are regarded as either **nominal** (category) or a **score** (figure). You need to be clear what type of data you are collecting as this will make a difference to how you analyse the data; it will also influence what conclusions can be drawn from the analysis. Certain statistical techniques that work with some kinds of data will not work with others. For further information see the next section: Basic understanding of statistics.

Essentially, quantitative data analysis involves analysing data collected that can be **numerically** counted or compared. It can initially describe the data in numbers and percentages and then involves some type of outcome measures, usually using a form of scoring or rating scale. This type of data can be manipulated and statistically analysed. Often the findings are represented visually in tables, graphs and charts to help you interpret and understand the results and make comparisons and see differences between groups.

Rating scales and ranking lists

There are a number of rating or scoring scales that are commonly used when undertaking quantitative research and either numbers or words (given a numerical score) can be used at varying anchor points on the scale. For example: when measuring the intensity of someone's pain there are several visual analogue scales (VAS) to indicate the level of pain. A VAS for pain consists of a straight line which is usually 10 cm in length and has number or word anchor points at each end to represent the extreme limits of pain (O'Hara, 1996). There are no words or numbers between the end points and a person marks or points to a place on the line to convey their level of pain at that present time. A VAS can be either a vertical or horizontal line (Figure 6.1).

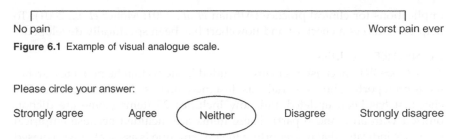

No pain   Worst pain ever

Figure 6.1 Example of visual analogue scale.

Please circle your answer:

Strongly agree   Agree   Neither   Disagree   Strongly disagree

Figure 6.2 Example of Likert scale.

Rating scales are often used to collect data concerning participant's opinions or views. The Likert scale is commonly used to find out how strongly or not a participant agrees with a statement or series of statements. Ideally, responses should be presented in a straight line rather than in multiple lines or columns, as this helps participants answer the questions more easily (Dillman, 2007) (Figure 6.2). It is also important to be consistent to avoid confusing participants.

Likert scales can include either even number of scores or uneven (as shown in Figure 6.2). Using a neutral score, such as 'Neither', 'Unsure', 'Don't know', gives participants the choice to remain neutral in their response and does not force them to choose. In the real world, there will always be a number of people who do not have either a positive or negative opinion or view on certain topics and including a neutral score represents these people. If an even number of scores is used and the neutral score is not included then this will force a participant to choose a response.

A ranking list allows participants to place their preferred choices in rank order and what they perceive are important. A researcher needs to make sure that the instructions are clear and concise so participants find it easy to answer and rank correctly. Cooper and Schindler (2008) have reported that ranking lists should not include more than seven options as too many will take too much effort to answer. An example of a ranking question is given in the section on Questionnaires in Chapter 4.

Consolidated Standards of Reporting Trials (CONSORT)

In the late 1980s and early 1990s, concerns were voiced that the quality of reports of randomised controlled trials (RCTs) was less than optimal (Pocock *et al.*, 1987; Altman & Doré, 1990). This instigated a consortium of representatives, involving medical journal editors, researchers, epidemiologists and methodologists, to undertake collaborative work to develop a valuable tool to assess the quality of RCT reports. This resulted in the development of the CONSORT Statement.

The CONSORT Statement is intended to improve the reporting of a RCT by researchers and it emphasises the importance of transparency to enable a person to understand and critique the study design, methods, findings and implications for clinical practice (Altman *et al.*, 2001; Moher *et al.*, 2001). To help this process a checklist and flowchart has been specifically developed.

CONSORT checklist

The CONSORT checklist originally included 22 items that helped a researcher focus on reporting how the trial was designed, analysed and interpreted. The checklist has been updated and now includes 25 items (some are dichotomised with an a and b part). These items are included because empirical evidence indicates that not reporting the information is associated with biased estimates of treatment effect, or because the information is essential to judge the reliability or relevance of the findings.

The CONSORT Statement 2010 checklist is intended to be accompanied with the explanatory document that facilitates its use. For more information, see Schulz *et al.* (2010) and Moher *et al.* (2010). The CONSORT statement gives revised recommendations for improving the quality of reports of parallel-group randomised trials. See weblink http://www.consort-statement.org and Table 6.1.

The CONSORT flowchart aims to demonstrate clearly the pathway participants take during a RCT. There is a free online resource that researchers can use to help them design a CONSORT flowchart (see weblink http://swolpin.cirg.washington.edu/CSD/ and Figures 6.3 and 6.4). Figure 6.4 uses the recommended CONSORT flowchart to demonstrate the progress mothers went through during the undertaking of a RCT that investigated the effectiveness of localised cooling treatments to alleviate perineal trauma (Steen & Marchant, 2007).

EQUATOR network is a website resource centre that developed from the work of CONSORT and other guideline development groups. This international network provides up-to-date resources related to health research reporting and is developing education and training facilities. (See weblink http://www.equator-network.org.)

Non-response bias

All quantitative research is subject to people not wanting to participate, withdrawing from the study and not returning questionnaires when enrolled in a study. This is a potential source of bias which a researcher has to acknowledge. It can reduce the effectiveness of the sample size and have an impact on the results found. Non-responders may differ in their characteristics to responders or they may not.

When you have non-respondents and you have tried to increase the rate of respondents, you will have to make a decision to analyse what data you have. So feasibly you can do both **intention to treat** and **complete case** analyses (on collected data only).

Intention to treat

To reduce analysis bias, all study participants should be included in the analyses of the groups to which they were randomised, regardless of whether

Table 6.1 CONSORT 2010 checklist of information to include when reporting a randomised trial. Reproduced under the creative commons agreement randomised trials. BMJ 2010;340:c332.

Section/topic	Item no	Checklist item	Reported on page no
Title and abstract			
	1a	Identification as a randomised trial in the title	
	1b	Structured summary of trial design, methods, results, and conclusions (for specific guidance see CONSORT for abstracts)	
Introduction			
Background and objectives	2a	Scientific background and explanation of rationale	
	2b	Specific objectives or hypotheses	
Methods			
Trial design	3a	Description of trial design (such as parallel, factorial) including allocation ratio	
	3b	Important changes to methods after trial commencement (such as eligibility criteria), with reasons	
Participants	4a	Eligibility criteria for participants	
	4b	Settings and locations where the data were collected	
Interventions	5	The interventions for each group with sufficient details to allow replication, including how and when they were actually administered	
Outcomes	6a	Completely defined pre-specified primary and secondary outcome measures, including how and when they were assessed	
	6b	Any changes to trial outcomes after the trial commenced, with reasons	
Sample size	7a	How sample size was determined	
	7b	When applicable, explanation of any interim analyses and stopping guidelines	
Randomisation:			
Sequence generation	8a	Method used to generate the random allocation sequence	
	8b	Type of randomisation; details of any restriction (such as blocking and block size)	
Allocation concealment mechanism	9	Mechanism used to implement the random allocation sequence (such as sequentially numbered containers), describing any steps taken to conceal the sequence until interventions were assigned	
Implementation	10	Who generated the random allocation sequence, who enrolled participants, and who assigned participants to interventions	
Blinding	11a	If done, who was blinded after assignment to interventions (for example, participants, care providers, those assessing outcomes) and how	
	11b	If relevant, description of the similarity of interventions	

Table 6.1 *Continued*

Section/topic	Item no	Checklist item	Reported on page no
Statistical methods	12a	Statistical methods used to compare groups for primary and secondary outcomes	
	12b	Methods for additional analyses, such as subgroup analyses and adjusted analyses	
Results			
Participant flow (a diagram is strongly recommended)	13a	For each group, the numbers of participants who were randomly assigned, received intended treatment and were analysed for the primary outcome	
	13b	For each group, losses and exclusions after randomisation, together with reasons	
Recruitment	14a	Dates defining the periods of recruitment and follow-up	
	14b	Why the trial ended or was stopped	
Baseline data	15	A table showing baseline demographic and clinical characteristics for each group	
Numbers analysed	16	For each group, number of participants (denominator) included in each analysis and whether the analysis was by original assigned groups	
Outcomes and estimation	17a	For each primary and secondary outcome, results for each group, and the estimated effect size and its precision (such as 95% confidence interval)	
	17b	For binary outcomes, presentation of both absolute and relative effect sizes is recommended	
Ancillary analyses	18	Results of any other analyses performed, including subgroup analyses and adjusted analyses, distinguishing pre-specified from exploratory	
Harms	19	All important harms or unintended effects in each group (for specific guidance see CONSORT for harms)	
Discussion			
Limitations	20	Trial limitations, addressing sources of potential bias, imprecision and, if relevant, multiplicity of analyses	
Generalisability	21	Generalisability (external validity, applicability) of the trial findings	
Interpretation	22	Interpretation consistent with results, balancing benefits and harms, and considering other relevant evidence	
Other information			
Registration	23	Registration number and name of trial registry	
Protocol	24	Where the full trial protocol can be accessed, if available	
Funding	25	Sources of funding and other support (such as supply of drugs), role of funders	

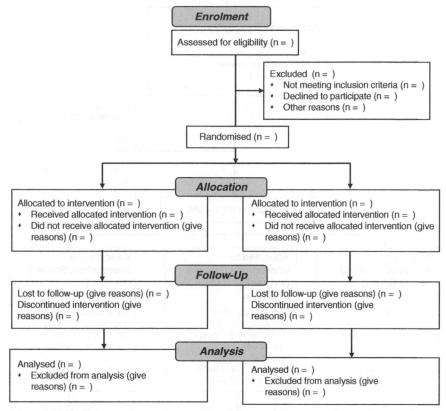

Figure 6.3 CONSORT 2010 flow diagram. Reproduced under the creative commons agreement randomised trials. BMJ 2010;340:c332.

they received the treatment allocated and completed the trial (Hollis & Campbell, 1999; Jahad, 2000).

Four things to remember:

- Participants are randomly assigned to a group.
- In the real world not everyone will get the treatment they have been allocated.
- 'Intention to treat' analysis means that statistical tests are carried out comparing the groups on the basis of the intended treatment even when this has not always occurred.
- Note – if we didn't do this we wouldn't be comparing groups that were randomly assigned (fundamental principle of RCT).

Inter-rater reliability
There will always be an element of subjectivity with how assessors will score or rate an observation but to try and reduce this to a minimum it is important

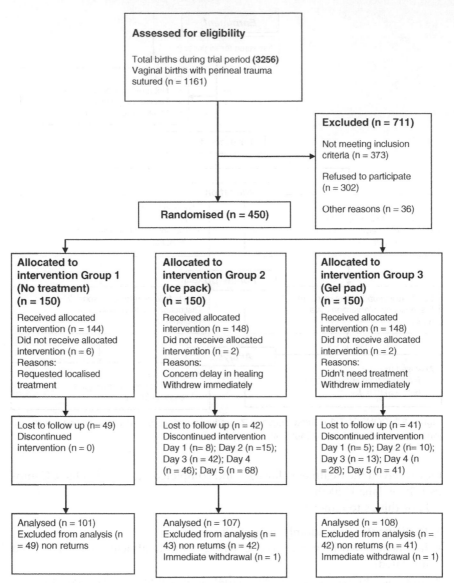

Figure 6.4 Flowchart of the progress through the phases of a randomised controlled trial.

that assessors have the knowledge, skills and experience to undertake the assessments and are able to use validated tools.

There will always be an element of subjectivity with how assessors will score or rate an observation but to try and reduce this to a minimum it is important that assessors have knowledge, skills and experience to undertake the assessments and are able to use validated tools. A researcher needs to consider the extent to which assessors measure things in the same way to increase the likelihood of agreement. Using validated assessment tools is helpful to reduce subjective levels of assessment and improve the credibility of the findings. The statistical test to measure inter-rater reliability between two assessors is the Cohen's Kappa.

A basic understanding of statistics

The main purpose of statistics is to accurately summarise the data into easily understandable information, as it is an extremely difficult task to make sense of large amounts of raw data that have not been prepared into some form of summary format.

Types of data

To begin with it is essential that you know what type of data you have to enable you to know what statistical test it is appropriate to use. There are four types of data you need to be able to recognise:

- **Discrete:** refers to whole numbers, i.e. singleton or multiple birth.
- **Continuous:** refers to a score being measured to the nearest unit.
- **Descriptive:** describes the data, i.e. frequencies, counts, percentages.
- **Inferential:** makes an inference to the general population at large.

There are also four levels of measurement (Table 6.2).

Levels of measurement

Nominal

This is sometimes referred to as naming data. This level of measurement is able to count things and place them into a category. Categories are based simply on names. It is recognised to be the lowest form of quantitative data analysis in the sense that it allows little by way of statistical manipulation compared to the other three levels of measurement.

   Examples: male/female; yes/no; good/bad; true/false.

Ordinal

This is similar to nominal data, as ordinal data are based on **counts of things** which are assigned to **specific categories**. However, what is important to remember is that the categories are in some form of rank order. Data in each

Table 6.2 Quantitative data.

Types of data	Levels of measurement
Discrete	Nominal
Continuous	Ordinal
Descriptive	Interval
Inferential	Ratio

category can be compared with data in other categories as being either lower or higher, more or less. It is also important to remember that rank order is all that can be inferred and ordinal data do not show the cause of the order or by how much the categories differ.

Example: a 5-point ordinal scale, such as intensity of pain:

None	Mild	Moderate	Severe	Very severe

Interval data

Interval data are similar to ordinal data in that they are also ranked but the specific categories ranked on a scale are proportionate. What that means is the correct distance between the categories is known and can be analysed more accurately. Similarly to ordinal data, you can analyse the data in terms of 'more than' or 'less than' but you can also say 'how much more' or 'how much less' and it allows for direct contrast and comparisons between the categories.

Example: calendar years are a good example and 10-year interval data is collected for years, i.e. 1970, 1980, 1990, 2000, 2010.

In the example above, interval data can compare the categories in terms of being an earlier or later decade of years, but can also compare an earlier or later time span interval. Interval data allows a researcher to use addition and subtraction (but not multiplication or division) to contrast the difference between various time periods. So, the difference between 1980 and 1990 can be directly compared with the difference between 2000 and 2010.

Ratio data

Ratio data are similar to interval data. The categories are proportionately ranked but what is important to remember is that these specific categories exist on a scale which has a **true zero** or an **absolute reference point**. For example, categories on a scale that concerns exact (precise) measures, such as distances, weight or temperature, gives rise to ratio data because the scale has a true zero point. In the previous interval data example (calendar years), years do not exist on such a scale as a true zero point does not denote the beginning of time.

When analysing ratio data it is important to remember that a researcher can compare and contrast the data for each category in terms of ratios using multiplication and division rather than being restricted to the use of addition and subtraction. Ratio data is the highest level of measurement for quantitative data in terms of how amenable it is to mathematical manipulation.

Descriptive statistics and inferential statistics

The main purpose of statistical analysis is to analyse the data collected from a sample so that inferences can be made to the population of interest. This will involve using descriptive and inferential statistics. Therefore, you will need to have a basic understanding of what these are and the common statistical tests you may come across when critiquing the evidence and undertaking a small scale research study yourself. The emphasis of the information is on the concepts of the statistics rather than calculations, as this will help you understand how results are reported in research articles. However, a few examples of how a test calculation can be carried out have been included to help you make sense of the data.

Descriptive statistics
Distribution
Normal distribution
Normal distribution is sometimes referred to as the Gaussian distribution that describes data that cluster around the mean. This standard distribution is a continuous probability distribution which is typically shown as bell-shaped with a peak at the mean (known as the bell curve) (Figure 6.5). A normal distribution is fundamental in statistics as many tests are based on the assumption that scores collected are distributed in a bell-shaped (normal) curve (Bowers, 2002).

Skewed distribution
A positively skewed distribution has a tail which is pulled in the positive direction. A negatively skewed distribution has a tail which is pulled in the negative direction (Figure 6.6).

Measures of central tendency
Once you have described your data in numbers and frequencies (how many), a good starting point to analyse the data is to use a measure of central tendency (mean, median, mode).

Average (or mean)
An example: a midwife books five women who are aged 22 years, 17 years, 24 years, 23 years and 29 years. The average maternal age is calculated as follows:

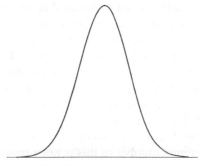

Figure 6.5 An example of a normal distribution.

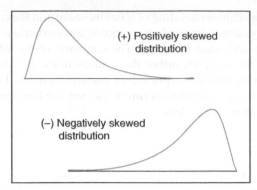

Figure 6.6 Skewed distribution.

The sum of all of the numbers (years) (22 + 17 + 24 + 23 + 29) = 115.
The total sum (115) is divided by the number of ages (5) to give an average (mean) age = 23 years.

The average is a descriptive statistic, which indicates a central or typical figure for a group of numbers.

Median
When you have a set of values, and need to obtain a figure which represents the central point, then arrange the numbers in order of size and choose the number which falls in the middle as being of typical value.

An example: if we have five babies weighing 3500 g, 4100 g, 2800 g, 3220 g, 3100 g, we arrange them in order of size (2800 g, 3100 g, 3220 g, 3500 g, 4100 g), and the median score is the value in the middle, i.e. the third score, 3220 g. If there had been six babies' weights to consider then you would take the weights of the third and fourth as two central numbers, 3220 g and 3500 g the median score would then be 3360 g (you could find this midpoint by adding the two numbers and then dividing by two, to find their average (or mean).

Mode
Mode is simply the value in any set of scores that occurs most often.

An example: have a look at the following set of numbers: 4, 6, 7, 7, 7, 8, 9, 9, 10. As the number 7 occurs most often (three times), 7 is the mode of these set of numbers. If one of the 7s disappeared we would have two 7s and two 9s; there would be two modes and this is known as bimodal.

This is a very useful statistic as it can be used to indicate a normal or usual figure. It is often used as the measure for an 'average person'; it is useful when the numbers in a distribution are not evenly spread around a central value. However, this measure of central tendency is not very helpful when there is a very low or high common number as this is not a true representation of the sample.

Measures of dispersion

Measures of dispersion are descriptive statistics used to qualify the word 'about' when looking at average scores. There are three commonly used measures of dispersion; the range, mean deviation and standard deviation.

Range

The range tells you over how many numbers altogether a distribution is spread. It is easily obtained by subtracting the smallest score from the largest. However, it isn't very reliable when your data set has extreme scores and this is why **quartile** measurements of dispersion are used. A distribution is divided into four equal parts or quartiles. The median is the average score that divides a distribution into two equal parts. Using this technique the scores in a distribution can be divided into quartiles. These quartiles give a better description of the dispersion in the data. The first quartile (Q1) is the midpoint between the lowest value and the second quartile (Q2) (at the median point) and the third quartile (Q3) is the midpoint between the highest value and the median (Q2).

Mean deviation

This measure of dispersion is not as commonly used as the range and standard deviation. The mean deviation is a number that indicates how much, on average, the scores in a distribution differ from a central point, the mean. It uses the absolute values of the deviation scores and not the squares of the deviation scores.

Standard deviation

Often shortened to sd, standard deviation is very similar to the mean deviation. It summarises an average distance of all the scores from the mean of a data set. It is, however, calculated in a different way. You need to take into account the signs (+ or −) of the deviations from the mean, and the result of this is that the mean deviation will always be zero. There is a solution to the problem. If you multiply two negative numbers together, you will get a positive result. The same applies to squaring a negative number (multiplying the number by itself).

This measure indicates just how much the word 'about' means for a set of figures and how widely the numbers scattered are. If one of these measures is used together with one of the measures of central tendency (averages), then the two summary numbers together will give an extremely concise and useful description of the particular distribution.

Hypothesis testing

When undertaking experimental research, a researcher will formulate a hypothesis to find out whether there is a relationship or differences between variables:

- **Alternative hypothesis** (H_1). There is a relationship between variables or there is a difference, and if a difference is found we confirm the alternative hypothesis.
- **Null hypothesis** (H_o). There is no actual relationship between variables or there is no difference, and if no significant difference is found we reject the null hypothesis.

A hypothesis can be:

- **one-tailed** – there is a relationship in one direction;
- **two-tailed** – there is a relationship between two variables in either direction.

Data are collected to either reject or accept an alternative or null hypothesis. However, there is always the possibility of error when testing a hypothesis. The rejecting or accepting of an alternative or null hypothesis and reporting the findings as significant when they are not and vice versa can occur. These are referred to as **type 1** and **type 2** errors:

- Type 1 (alpha error) is the error of rejecting a null hypothesis and stating there is no difference between variables being tested when in fact there is a difference.
- Type 2 (beta error) is the error of not rejecting a null hypothesis when there is actually a false result and consequently accepting there is no difference when there is.

Sample size

The general population is too large for the researcher to attempt to recruit everyone and a representative sample is carefully chosen as a sample. The sample reflects the characteristics of the population chosen.

Sampling methods are classified as either **probability** or **non-probability**. Probability sampling is any method of sampling that involves some form of random selection (Walliman, 2005). In contrast, non-probability sampling does not involve random selection (Hicks, 1996). Probability methods include simple random, stratified random, systematic and cluster sampling, whereas non-probability methods include a non-random sample, such as convenience sampling, quota sampling or snowball sampling.

Random sampling gives each person in the population targeted a calculable probability of being selected for inclusion in the study (Casey & Devane, 2010). It is important to note that random sampling relates to the method of sampling and not the resulting sample (Bowling, 2009). For probability sampling standard formulae can be applied to ascertain the precision expected from a random sample of a certain size. Usually, some prior estimate of the population parameter of interest is needed to obtain a value for the sample size.

Sampling error

All sample results are likely to be affected by sampling errors and the mean of a sample will not be exactly the same as the total population mean; this difference is known as sampling error. When undertaking a research study, a sample of participants in one study can differ when compared to a similar sample selected if the study were replicated. Basically, what this means is that no sample is completely representative of the population being studied.

An advantage of probability sampling, however, is that sampling error can be calculated. Sampling error is the degree to which a sample might differ from the population at large. When inferring to the population, results are reported plus (+) or minus (−) the sampling error. In non-probability sampling, the degree to which the sample differs from the population remains unknown.

Odds ratio

Odds ratio (OR) is a descriptive statistic that measures the ratio of the odds of an event or condition occurring in one group to the odds of it occurring in another group. It is sometimes used as a form of analysis in clinical trials and the groups compared would be the experimental versus the control group. It measures effect size and describes the strength of a relationship. Relationships are measured by the difference from 1.0 and an OR < 1.0 indicates a negative relationship and an OR > 1.0 indicates a positive relationship. An OR of 1.0 indicates that the odds are equally likely to occur in both groups. It treats two variables being compared symmetrically.

An example: in a sample of 100 primiparous women, 60 disclose they smoke at the booking appointment and in a sample of 100 multiparous women, 40 disclose they smoke. The odds of a primiparous woman smoking are 60 to 40 or 6:4, while the odds of a multiparous woman smoking are 40 to 60 or 4:6.

$$\frac{0.6/0.4}{0.4/0.6} = \frac{0.6 \times 0.6}{0.4 \times 0.4} = \frac{0.36}{0.16} = 2.25$$

In this example primiparous women are $60/40 = 1.5$ times more likely to smoke than multiparous women but have 2.25 times the odds.

Relative risk

Relative risk (RR) relates to the risk of an event (or developing a condition) relative to exposure. It is a risk ratio of the probability of the event/condition occurring in the exposed group versus a non-exposed group.

An example: the probability of developing pre-eclampsia among pregnant women with a BMI > 30 is 25% and in women with a BMI < 30 is 1%. See table below:

| | Pre-eclampsia | |
	Present	Absent
Women BMI > 30	a	b
Women BMI < 30	c	d

$$RR = \frac{a/(a+b)}{c/(c+d)} = \frac{25/100}{1/100} = 25$$

Pregnant women with a BMI > 30 would be 25 times more likely to develop pre-eclampsia than women with a BMI < 30.

Confidence intervals

Confidence intervals are often used to inform the reader of the range of values in which we are likely to find the true value of the population parameter. That is the parameter value resides between its upper and lower confidence limits, with say 95% confidence. In other words, under many repeat samplings 95% of the confidence intervals generated will contain the value of the parameter. Of course we don't know if our single sample confidence interval does or whether it is one of the 5% which do not. The most frequently used confidence interval (CI) is the 95% but sometimes 99% can be used.

An example: a group of pregnant women with hypertension receive an anti-hypertensive drug; we measure their systolic BP pre and post having the drug. The result shows a mean fall of 12 mmHg but this value could be influenced by chance. A 95% CI for our 12 mmHg was 8–16 mmHg; this means we are 95% confident that the population mean is in that range. We can make a scientific claim that the drug is effective at lowering blood pressure in this population.

Numbers needed to treat

Numbers needed to treat (NNR) relates to the number of patients who need to be treated to prevent one bad outcome, in others words the numbers needed to be treated so one will benefit from the treatment. It is used as a measure for evaluating the effectiveness of a treatment or intervention.

An example: a randomised controlled trial which compared continuous versus interrupted suturing for perineal repair reported that a continuous repair technique can prevent one woman in six from having pain at 10 days (Kettle *et al.*, 2002). This trial also reported that using the more rapidly absorbed polyglactin 910 suture material when compared with standard poly-glactin 910 material avoided the need for suture removal up to 3 months postpartum for one in ten women sutured.

Inferential statistics: statistical tests

A power calculation

The sample size for a trial needs to be planned carefully and at the outset it is important to have assistance from a statistician. A study should be large enough to have the power of detecting statistically significant difference and a clinically important difference, if such a difference exists.

Elements of the sample size calculation are (Campbell *et al.*, 1995):

* the estimated outcomes in each group (which implies the clinically important target difference between the intervention groups);
* the alpha (type 1) error level;
* the statistical power, or the beta (type 2) error level;
* and, for continuous outcomes, the standard deviation of the measurements.

A researcher needs to indicate how the sample size was determined and calculated. The primary outcome on which the calculation was based should be stated and all the quantities used in the calculation and what the sample size per group should be. It is preferable to quote the proposed results of each group rather than the expected difference between the groups. In addition, details should be given of any allowance made for attrition during the study.

An example: power calculation used by Dahlen (2007) for a trial that was investigating the reduction of perineal trauma and improved perineal comfort during and after childbirth:

* The primary outcome was perineal suturing following childbirth.
* The process involved using birth records from the previous 7 years
* It was estimated that 25% of all women required no perineal suturing.
* To detect a reduction of 10% in suturing with a power of 80% (alpha = 0.05, two-sided test), 694 women needed to be randomised.
* This was considered to be clinically significant.
* 1047 women were asked to participate in the trial, 717 were randomised.

A useful resource you can register for free to assist you to undertake power calculations is GPower*3 which is a statistical software programme that allows high-precision power and sample size analyses (Camacho-Sandoval, 2007). Most statisticians, however, have software to do this task.

See weblink http://www.psycho.uni-duesseldorf.de/abteilungen/aap/gpower3/.

Parametric and non-parametric tests

* **Parametric tests** make the assumption that the data are drawn from a normal distribution. The quantitative data are measured on an interval or ratio scale (i.e. real numbers, height, weight, temperature) and the tests also make use of parameters such as the mean and sd.
* **Non-parametric tests** make no assumptions at all about the population from which the data are drawn. Knowledge of parameters is not necessary and generally they are easier to learn and apply. The most commonly used are chi-square and Mann–Whitney *U* test.

What does statistical significance mean?

It means that you are sure that the statistic is reliable. It does not mean the finding is clinically important or that it has any decision-making usefulness. Statistical significance is used in comparative (experimental studies). It is a useful measure to compare two or more groups to see if there are any differences between groups or is it just a chance finding. Statistical tests tell us how likely this is and this probability expressed as a p-value: p-values of $p < 0.05$, $p < 0.01$, $p < 0.001$ are commonly used for statistical significance of differences between variables. The smaller the p-value, i.e. $p < 0.001$, the less likely it is that the result has occurred by chance. The choice of $p < 0.05$ (5% level) is conventionally taken as the error level required to declare a positive result (there is a difference between groups).

Less than $p < 0.05$ can state that there is a statistical significant difference at the 5% level. A p-value of 0.05 means 5% probability, there are 5 chances in 100 (or a 1 in 20 chance) the finding would occur by chance. A 5% probability (cut-off) point means that if the result is less than the 5% (cut-off) level then it is deemed to be statistically significant and there is a statistical difference between the groups.

t-test and analysis of variance

The t-test and analysis of variance (ANOVA) are parametric tests. The t-test measures whether the means of two groups are significantly different from each other. (Mann–Whitney U test is the non-parametric equivalent.) A t-test could be used to measure the mean length of labour of primigravida and multigravida. ANOVA does essentially the same thing with more groups.

An example of the t-test being used was to analyse the mean improvement of 95 midwives' and 17 obstetricians' knowledge-base of cardiotocography and acid–base balance in an RCT undertaken by Beckley *et al.* (2000). This trial investigated the development and evaluation of a computer-assisted teaching programme for intrapartum fetal monitoring. The results demonstrated that the teaching programme was effective in improving knowledge. The mean improvement from test 1 to test 2 was 19.4% (95% CI 16.5–22.3%) $p < 0.0001$, paired t-test for early group and 4.3% (95% CI 1.6–7.0%) $p = 0.003$, paired t-test for late group.

Correlation coefficient tests

The Pearson's is a statistic that is used to show the degree of 'linear relationship' between variables that have been measured on interval or ratio scales. It is symbolised as r. For example, a correlation between a pregnant woman's weight and height measurement could be calculated. It is the most common correlation statistic used but there are also others such as Kendall's and Spearman's that are used when variables are in rank order on an ordinal scale.

Kendall's correlation would be used when the ranks of the ordered categories are not treated as interval scales. Spearman's, symbolised as r_s, assesses how well a (monotonic) relationship between two variables can be described.

If there are no repeated data values a perfect correlation of +1 or −1 can be achieved when each of the variables are in perfect monotone of the other. For example, is there a relationship between midwifery knowledge and age? A sample of midwives could be given a test relating to midwifery knowledge and then be ranked by their ages and scores. A Spearman's test can calculate if there is a relationship between these two rankings.

Kendall's coefficient of concordance is a non-parametric test used to measure the level of agreement among sets of rankings. It is symbolised as W which can range from 0 (no agreement) to 1.0 (total agreement). For example, if you wanted to see how much 10 pregnant women agreed (in concord) about the usefulness of a number of pregnancy books this statistic would calculate this.

Chi-square test (χ^2)

Chi-square test (χ^2) is a non-parametric test and deals with frequencies data. It is a useful statistical test, that can tell you whether the pattern of observations you have collected is significantly different from what you might expect by chance. It is important to note that this test can only be used in situations where the groups are mutually exclusive, e.g. primigravida or multigravida, smoker or non-smoker.

An example: is there statistically significant difference between the observed (actual) frequencies and the expected or hypothesised (null hypothesis). The frequencies and test significance of two variables are presented in Table 6.3 (cross-tabulation).

Degrees of freedom (df) relates to the number of values free to vary when computing a statistic. This number is required when calculating a chi-square test. See the chi-square test example given. Basically, in this example the df are computed by multiplying the number of rows minus 1 ($R - 1$) times the number of columns minus 1 ($C - 1$). So, $df = (R - 1)(C - 1)$. The example shows a 2×2 table: it has two rows and two columns: the $df = (R - 1)(C - 1) = (2 - 1)(2 - 1) = 1 \times 1 = 1$. The more categories the variables are divided into the higher the df will be.

Mann–Whitney U Test

The Mann–Whitney U test is a non-parametric test for assessing whether two independent samples of observations come from the same distribution. It is used when data are measured on an ordinal scale (in rank order). See Table 6.4 and Figure 6.7.

Kruskal–Wallis test

The Kruskal–Wallis test is a non-parametric test of statistical significance. It is used when testing more than two independent samples and is similar to the Mann–Whitney U test.

An example: in a RCT, women in groups 1 and 2 overall rated their perineal care to be 'Good' whilst group 3 rated it to be 'Very good' to 'Excellent' (see

Table 6.3 Test of independence. (Null) hypothesis: smoking mothers are not affected by having a second baby, i.e. smoking and having babies are independent factors and not inter-related.

Observed	Non-smokers	Smokers	Totals
1st-time mothers	19	23	42
2nd time	42	16	58
Totals	61	39	100

Expected frequencies	Non-smokers	Smokers	Totals
1st-time mothers	26	16	42
2nd time	35	23	58
Totals	61	39	100
# Rows	2		
# Columns	2		
Degrees of freedom	1		
χ^2	8.48		
p-value	0.00360		

Significance:
If p-value >0.05 accept hypothesis, and conclude that the factors are independent and the results could be produced by chance
If p-value <0.05 reject hypothesis and conclude that the factors are inter-related and the results are not produced by chance

Table 6.4 Pain during use of cooling treatment – day 1 (Steen, 2004).

	Worse	Same	Less	Stopped	Statistical significance
Ice pack	5 (5%)	23 (21.4%)	67 (63%)	4 (4%)	p = 0.0015
Gel pad	2 (2%)	12 (11%)	75 (69%)	14 (13%)	

Table 6.5 and Figure 6.8). This was statistically significant (p = 0.0001, df = 2), Kruskal–Wallis test (Steen & Marchant, 2001).

Cohen's kappa

Cohen's kappa measures the agreement between two raters/assessors assessing a number of units (Cohen, 1960). This statistical test calculates the proportion of units where there is agreement and the proportion of units expected to agree by chance.

The equation for κ is

$$\kappa = \frac{p - p_e}{1 - p_e}$$

p is the proportion of observed agreement among the two raters/assessors overall and p_e is the hypothetical probability of chance agreement using the observed row and column marginals to calculate the probabilities of each observer randomly choosing the same category under the assumption of

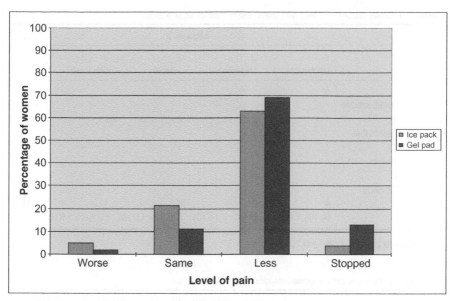

Figure 6.7 Self-assessed pain during use of the cooling device – day 1.

Table 6.5 Maternal satisfaction with perineal care (Steen & Marchant, 2001).

	Poor	Fair	Good	Very good	Excellent
Group 1 No treatment	0	16 (16%)	49 (49%)	19 (19%)	16 (16%)
Group 2 Ice pack	1 (1%)	23 (23%)	39 (38%)	26 (25%)	13 (13%)
Group 3 Gel pad	2 (19%)	5 (5%)	23 (22%)	44 (41%)	32 (30%)

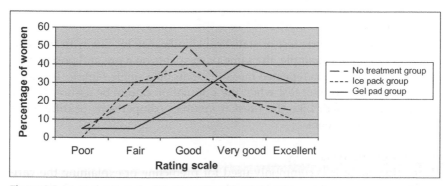

Figure 6.8 Level of maternal satisfaction with perineal care.

Table 6.6 Cross-tabulation: two midwives' estimates of scar tissue.

		Midwife 2				Total
		1 *Undetectable*	*2* *Detectable*	*3* *Visible*	*4* *Obvious*	
Midwife 1	1 Undetectable	4				4
	2 Detectable		2	2		4
	3 Visible			1		1
	4 Obvious				1	1
Total		4	2	3	1	10
P_{i-j}		$(4/10) \times (4/10)$	$(2/10) \times (4/10)$	$(3/10) \times (1/10)$	$(1/10) \times (1/10)$	0.28

$\kappa = (8/10 - 0.28)/(1 - 0.28) = 0.7222$

Table 6.7 Cohen's kappa – statistical test (Steen, 2004).

		Value	*Asymp. std. error*	*Approx. T*	*Approx. sig.*
Measure of agreement	Kappa	0.722	0.161	4.007	0.000
No of valid cases		10			

independence. If the raters/assessors totally agree then $\kappa = 1$, if the raters/assessors only agree by chance then $\kappa = 0$.

The number agreeing and disagreeing can be seen in a cross-tabulation table, just like that used as in a chi-square test of independence, i.e. by row and column totals, (marginal frequencies) from which the proportions can be calculated.

An example: two midwives' estimates of perineal scar tissue (Steen, 2004). See Tables 6.6 and 6.7.

There are extensions for more than two raters and also ways to take the size of disagreements into account.

Wilcoxon test

This is a non-parametric test of statistical significance for use with two cor-related samples, for example, the same participants on a pre and post test, or it can also be used with repeated measurements on a single sample. It is used as an alternative to the *t*-test when the population cannot be assumed to be normally distributed. Like the *t*-test it involves comparisons of differences between measurements.

Regression analysis

Regression analysis is commonly used for predicting or explaining the vari-ability of a dependent variable from information about one or more independent variables. It gives an indication of how the typical value of the dependent variable changes when any one of the independent variables is varied and when other independent variables are held fixed.

Logistic regression is used for the prediction of the probability of occurrence of an event by fitting the data to a logistic curve. It makes use of several predictor variables that may be either numerical or categorical.

An example: Downe *et al.* (2004) used logistic regression analysis for potential confounding variables due to a large variation in maternal weight between randomised groups in a trial that investigated whether the rate of instrumental birth in first-time mothers using epidural analgesia was affected by maternal position in the passive second stage of labour. The dependent variable was mode of delivery and nine independent variables were included in the regression analysis, these were: maternal age at booking, BMI at booking, use of oxytocin drugs in labour, position of baby's head and its relation to the mother's ischial spines on full dilation of cervix, maternal position in the passive second stage of labour, length of active second stage of labour, decision to have an instrumental delivery, total dose of local anaesthetic prior to top-up for instrumental delivery. Only the position of the baby's head at full dilation affected the risk of instrumental delivery, $p = 0.4$, OR 2.7; maternal weight did not have any effect.

Fisher's Exact Test

A statistical test known as the Fisher's Exact Test may have to be used when the analysis involves a small sample. It is used mainly in 2×2 frequency tables when the expected frequency is too small to rely on the use of the chi-square test.

An excellent resource which is available online is *Statistics Guide for Research Grant Applicants* (Authors, in alphabetical order, JM Bland, BK Butland, JL Peacock, J Poloniecki, F Reid, P Sedgwick). See weblink http://www-users.york.ac.uk/~mb55/guide/guide.htm.

Summary

This chapter has focused on how to make sense of the data. One of the most important steps in the research process is the analysis of gathered data. Basic principles of data analysis have been introduced and specific sections relating to qualitative and quantitative data analysis methods have been covered in detail. Examples of both qualitative and quantitative midwifery data analysis methods have been included to assist midwives and students to learn and consolidate their knowledge and skills.

Qualitative data analysis is a creative but time-consuming process that needs to be systematic and transparent. Thematic analysis, data analysis frameworks, some useful resources and software have been suggested in this chapter to help midwives and students undertake a qualitative data analysis.

In addition, a basic understanding of statistics, that has covered both descriptive and inferential concepts and some statistical calculations, has been included in this chapter. This information is necessary to help midwives and students link the type of data collected with the appropriate statistical test required to analyse a specific type of data. Examples relating to midwifery research and practice have been given to assist midwives and student to understand how statistics can be used within the profession. Useful resources and statistical software packages to help analyse quantitative data have also been included in this chapter.

It is envisaged that midwives and students will have increased their confidence and competences to analyse both qualitative and quantitative data after reading this chapter. Working through the examples given will assist midwives and students to gain analytical skills and this will help them in their understanding of data. It is important that midwives and students disseminate their research findings and the next chapter covers this research activity.

7 Research dissemination

Introduction

This final chapter will focus on writing skills and will stress the importance of disseminating evidence whether the findings are positive or not. Guidance on how to write a research dissertation and to write a paper will be explored and discussed. Midwives and students will be encouraged to not stop there and to go on and publish their research study and present a conference paper. Useful resources and information on becoming a researcher will be further discussed. It is envisaged that some student midwives will be inspired to continue and develop further research skills. Once qualified some may even go on to undertake further midwifery research!

Learning outcomes

By the end of this final chapter midwives and students:

- will have developed some scholarly writing skills;
- will be able to write a research report successfully;
- will be inspired to write a paper for publication;
- will be inspired to write and submit a conference paper;
- will gain some presentation skills and the confidence to present a paper.

The dissertation

Your dissertation is a learning opportunity to study independently and examines your ability to educate yourself. However, there is '*a lot to learn and not much time to learn it*' (Walliman, 2004). It is essential that you receive guidance and support but you need to take responsibility and actions to meet your own learning needs that will enable you to successfully achieve this task.

At the commencement of your dissertation module you will be guided as to what you have to achieve within a specified time period. Usually, at

The Handbook of Midwifery Research, First Edition. Mary Steen and Taniya Roberts.
© 2011 Mary Steen and Taniya Roberts. Published 2011 by Blackwell Publishing Ltd.

undergraduate level the dissertation is a double module and this reflects the amount of study that is expected from you. It is an excellent opportunity for you to develop both personally and professionally. Initially, you will need to attend some formal sessions and an overview of the **research process, plan of work** and **how to write a research proposal** will be covered. You will need to demonstrate theoretical and practical aspects of how you would undertake a research study. You will be self-directed and expected to write a research proposal of about 8000–10000 words. Postgraduate studies require more in-depth knowledge and understanding of research; it will involve the actual undertaking of a research study as full or partial requirement of a Master's, MPhil or PhD qualification and is a substantial piece of work. The word length can vary slightly depending on different university requirements and can be anything from 15000–25000 words for a Master's, MPhil thesis and from 60000–80000 words for a PhD. In addition, some universities are now offering a taught or professional PhD programme of study and this may be an option for you to consider.

Whether you are doing undergraduate or postgraduate study you will need to decide relatively quickly on a topic you would like to research and consider what research question you want to ask.

Make sure you contact your allocated supervisor early and plan supervisory meetings as this will help you learn and monitor your progress carefully. Always try to have your research proposal peer reviewed as this may offer you suggestions. If possible, ask an experienced researcher for some advice. You should give yourself plenty of time to write a draft copy first. Any amendments or further work required can then be undertaken. You may find it helpful to include this task in your plan of work (Figure 7.1).

Service user involvement

Consider how you are going to involve service users and you could consider the RDInfo's recommended four stages of the research process for user involvement mentioned earlier to guide you in:

- setting the research agenda;
- developing the proposal;
- during the conduct of the project;
- disseminating results.

Guidance on supervision

It is your responsibility to arrange to meet with your academic supervisor. Ideally the initial meeting should be within the first 4–6 weeks of you commencing your dissertation module or postgraduate thesis. Do not put it off, contacting your supervisor should be on your list of things to do; nowadays, an email seems to be one of the quickest ways to communicate with supervisors or you can make a telephone call with the option of leaving a voicemail if the call is unanswered. If you can, give a few possible dates of your

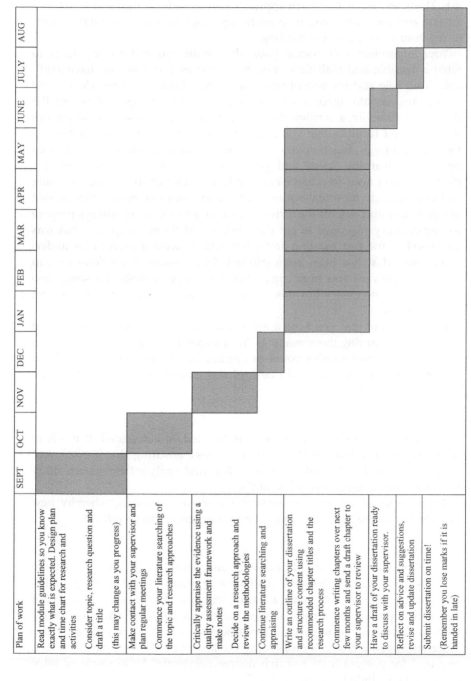

Figure 7.1 Plan of work – undergraduate dissertation.

availability so a mutual time can be arranged. Prior to the meeting make some notes of what topic ideas you have and what question(s) you would like to ask. Think about what research approach you consider is the most suitable to answer any question(s) you are considering. Ask your supervisor if they want to see your work prior to a meeting.

Your supervisor will discuss your ideas with you and guide you as to what is feasible and realistic within the resources and time you have available. Your role and the role of your supervisor should be made clear at the outset. You should agree a schedule for further meetings and record the dates and times in a written diary or electronically. Most mobile phones have calendar facilities that you can make use of and alert you to dates and times of meetings. Together you can devise a plan of work which will focus upon your learning needs and your research proposal/study. Logically, plan what you need to achieve and produce a **time chart** for your learning and research activities. Make sure you have the submission date highlighted in your diary and tick off the activities as you achieve them. Always prepare for supervisory meetings to get the most out of them, recap on what was discussed at the last meeting and what actions were agreed to be undertaken and what has been accomplished. Circumstances not foreseen can sometimes prevent you from completing your agreed goals and some flexibility will be necessary but this is the real world and you can always get back on track.

It is important that you keep a written record of the main points covered and discussed during these meetings. Your supervisor will also keep a record of the meetings and monitor your learning and research activities. Ethical and research governance issues will be explored as well as confidentiality and academic integrity.

The research process
The research proposal needs to be well planned and designed. It needs to incorporate every facet of the research process, ensuring that a systematic course of action is followed to access, collect and analyse the research study findings. Box 7.1 gives an outline of this.

These series of actions demonstrate the research process, whereby new knowledge can be generated or existing information can be refined.

Guidance on the structure of a research proposal
Midwifery research is steadily evolving and covers many areas of interest utilising both quantitative and qualitative approaches and methodologies. Most research proposals have a basic structure but, depending on your research approach and methodology, there will be some variation to the content. If you are an undergraduate student your dissertation is a written assignment and a research proposal so the layout is slightly different to that required for postgraduate research degree proposals. An example of what needs to be included is given in Box 7.2.

Box 7.1 An outline of the research process.

- Decide on the research question. What is the information that you want to find out about?
- Perform a literature review to find out if the research has already been conducted (the exception being grounded theory).
- If the research has already been completed, consider if your research is needed or do you need to modify the question.
- Decide on how best to go about collecting the information to answer your research question.
- Carefully plan your research design to incorporate the most appropriate methodology.
- Do ensure that you utilise the following correctly and discuss them in your proposal:
  - paradigm;
  - quantitative or qualitative approach;
  - methodology (experimental, e.g. RCT, or non-experimental, e.g. survey; phenomenology, e.g. Husserlian);
  - hypothesis or question;
  - ethical considerations (ethical approval, consent to the clinical area, informed consent from the study participants etc.);
  - sample and recruitment;
  - data collection methods;
  - data analysis methods;
  - consider costings of the project;
  - decide how you are going to discuss and present the findings/results;
  - the implications for midwifery practice;
  - decide how you plan on disseminating the findings of your research study.

Research degree – proposals

Higher education institutions set criteria to be met by applicants to undertake an MPhil or PhD research degree. Usually, a 'good' first degree, i.e. a 1st or 2.1 and if students have a 2.2 degree, then this is acceptable if you have completed a Master's degree. Your degree should ideally be in an area relevant to your proposed research. However, there is some flexibility and many universities will consider applicants on a case-by-case basis. Some universities ask you to complete an application form which includes a précis section to complete about your proposed research and a personal statement section to find out why you want to undertake this research. Normally, an applicant will have an interview and may have to attend a pre-registration course before being accepted. The aim of the interview is to see whether there is expertise available to supervise and support you to undertake the research and that you

Box 7.2 The dissertation: guidance for writing a research proposal.

Title: this is a statement not the research question and should include the type of study, the subject and population of interest.

Abstract: this can be structured or unstructured and gives a summary of the research proposed.

Background/Rationale: sets the scene and states why this research is needed. You can refer to evidence to support your claim and also justify the research approach you have chosen.

Literature review: you need to do an in-depth literature search relating to your topic and also on your chosen research approach and methodology, so you can write a balanced argument to support your research proposal. You will find using a quality assessment framework to critique the research useful as this will assist you to focus on the strengths and weaknesses of the research study and evidence reported. Make notes and summarise important findings, gaps in the literature and inconclusive evidence.

Research question: your literature review will assist you to structure a research question that needs to be asked.

Aim: you need to state clearly what it is you intend to do. You may also want to include some objectives about how you are going to achieve this.

Methodology: you need to describe and discuss the research paradigm and approach you have chosen (quantitative or qualitative), and then give details and information about the methodology you have chosen. You will need to justify why this methodology is 'fit for purpose' and why you have chosen it over all other methodologies.

Sample and setting: the sample size will depend on your research approach and methodology. You will need to discuss how the sample will be recruited and also the setting where the research will be undertaken.

Pilot study: this also depends on your research approach and methodology; you definitely need one if you have chosen an experimental design. It is also good practice to test out your study design and any evaluating tools so problems can be rectified before the main study is commenced.

Reliability and credibility: you will need to demonstrate that you have considered the reliability and validity of your study (quantitative) or the credibility and trustworthiness of your study (qualitative) and how will you ensure this.

Data collection: you will have to describe and discuss the data collection method and tool(s) you will be using to gather and record data. You need to justify why this method and tool is appropriate and link it to the research approach and methodology.

Data analysis: again, this will depend of your research approach and methodology. You will need to demonstrate how you intend to analyse and present your findings. If you have chosen quantitative research then include descriptive and inferential statistics, any computer software packages and seek advice from a statistician. If you have chosen qualitative research, you need to discuss how emerging themes will be developed, any framework to be used to assist in undertaking a thematic analysis and if any computer software packages will be used.

Ethical considerations: you will need to consider and discuss ethical issues and demonstrate that potential participants are able to make an informed consent, are not put at unnecessary risk, that benefits outweigh any risks and participants are aware that they can withdraw at anytime without their care being affected in any way.

Research governance: this basically means how you are going to manage and monitor the research. You will need to consider how you are going to involve participants, how you are going to gain access to them and permission to do so. You will also need to consider health and safety issues for the participant and you as the researcher.

Costing: you will need to include an estimate of all costs for your proposed study. This should include your time, travel, any equipment such as audio-tape recorder, computer software packages, stationery and stamps.

Plan of work: you will need to include details of your proposed research which can include phases, months and milestones. A calendar timetable or Gantt chart are useful aids.

Implications for practice: you will need to discuss the potential benefits of your research to midwifery, maternity services, women, their babies and their families.

Dissemination: you will need to consider how you are going to disseminate your research findings, submit a publication, give a conference paper, a report to ethics committee, maternity unit, etc.

Professional considerations: you will need to consider implications for professional conduct and adhere to guidance, codes and regulations.

Appendices: you will need to include copies of covering letters, to be sent to midwifery managers, general practitioners and potential participants (anonymised), information leaflets, consent forms and data collection tools (questionnaire, interview schedule). In addition, include a page indicating where the curriculum vitae of the researcher would be.

List of references and bibliography: you will need to include all references that have been used in your research proposal and a bibliography of all the sources of information you have referred to. Make sure you check your references and that all are listed; use the referencing system advocated by the university.

Table 7.1 Basic time plan – template.

Month	1	2	3	4	5	6	7	8	9	10	11	12
Phase 1												
Phase 2												
Phase 3												
Phase 4												
Milestones												

have the ability to complete the research degree. The availability of resources and funding will also be reviewed. If you are accepted you will need to prepare a research proposal. Generally this will need to include:

- a title (short and long version);
- lay summary or abstract (approximately 250–300 words);
- introduction (setting the scene) (main body approximately 2500 words);
- background (discusses literature and rationale as to why the research is needed);
- methods (research approach and methodology);
- ethical considerations;
- health and safety (research governance);
- costing;
- references.

Adapted from: *Guide to Postgraduate Research Degrees (MPhil & PhD)* (2010) University of Chester.

Sinclair (2008, p. 3) defines midwifery research as:

> a rigorous process of inquiry that aims to provide knowledge of, and insights into, the efficacy and effectiveness of midwifery practice; its effects on women, babies, parents, family and society. It includes research on the education and training of midwives, the use of information and communication technologies, the organisation and delivery of maternity services and employment conditions and terms affecting midwives' working lives.

When undertaking research it is helpful to design a time plan including the phases, months and milestones that are proposed to assist the successful completion of the research (see Tables 7.1 and 7.2).

Writing skills

Writing is acknowledged as a powerful tool for learning as well as for communicating (Yinger, 1985). All research has implications for education, policy, management and practice. It is essential that you develop good writing skills and techniques to disseminate your research as this will promote learning

Table 7.2 An example of a time plan to undertake an RCT to investigate the use of moxibustion for turning a breech presentation.

Phases	Months	Milestones
Phase 1: preparation		
Ethical application and R & D approval	6 months	NHS Research Clinical Governance Framework (Department of Health, 2005)
Project Steering Group		Project Steering Group selected
Raising awareness of RCT		Design, posters, leaflets to raise awareness In-service education and training
Preparing for RCT	4 months	Design research protocol, information leaflet, consent form, diaries, questionnaires, coding for analysis, order moxi sticks
Phase 2: the RCT		
Recruitment of participants	12 months	Randomise xxx women to two arms (xxx experimental group vs xxx control group)
The trial		Demonstrate procedure for moxibustion
Coordinate, supervise		Be visible, accessible, available for queries Contact number for any daily problems
Collecting data		Completion of semi-structured questionnaires and diaries
Monitoring of the trial		Monthly meetings for core planning team Annual meeting, steering group and users
Phase 3: analysis of data		
Entering data into SPSS software		On-going during trial, cross-checking for error
Using SPSS software	12 months	Research consultant and statistican
Confidentiality and storage of data		In accordance with NHS Governance Framework (Department of Health, 2005)
Phase 4: dissemination of findings		
Sharing the findings with peers, users	2 months	Report to funders, publications, conference papers, editorials, NHS Trust Newsletter and website, local newspapers

within the profession and inform future care that is based on evidence. Your writing skills will have improved whilst undertaking a midwifery degree or continual professional education but by writing articles you will further develop your writing skills. Remember to vary the length of sentences as this helps to emphasise important points and ideas. A long sentence followed by a short sentence will direct the reader to an important issue. New paragraphs should be introduced when you are describing and discussing a new idea or concept. Proof-reading is very important as this will assist you to detect any grammar, punctuation and typing errors. Ideally, get a colleague or friend to proof-read your article as you often can suffer from 'writer's blindness'. In particular check for words that confuse most people such as 'affect' and 'effect', as these are often incorrectly used. Affect is a verb and means 'have an impact on', for example 'this will affect your health and well-being', whereas 'effect' is usually a noun, for example 'this had a good effect on health and well-being'. To effect means 'to bring about or cause', for example 'to effect a change in maternity care policy'.

Unfortunately, time constraints and clinical practice demands can make it difficult for midwives and students to write and publish their research findings or give a conference presentation. You may think, why bother, when you know it is a time-consuming task and it can be a lengthy process for the research findings to then filter into the clinical practice setting. Remember the passion you had to undertake the research study at the outset! You made a commitment and designed a plan of dissemination to gain ethics approval: you need to see it through to the end. This is the final hurdle. Just think of the effort you have put into this so far, what you have achieved and the new knowledge and skills you have acquired. Believe in yourself and your ability.

It is vitally important that every effort is made to disseminate the findings of research whether there is evidence of groundbreaking new knowledge and clear benefits to women, their babies and families, or the exact opposite. There may be no new knowledge and no clear benefits identified or even some evidence that an element of practice is in fact detrimental to the target group.

Writing styles
Writing in the first, second or third person
When writing in the first person, 'I', 'me', 'we', 'my' or 'our' are used and refer to the person who is speaking. Generally, you would use this style when writing personal reflections or a personal statement. A diary, personal journal and reflective assignments would be written in the first person.

When writing in the second person, 'you' is used and it refers to the person who is listening. This narrative style is not often used in literature. The second person has been used occasionally in this book to enable the authors to engage with you and get some important points across.

When writing in the third person, 'it',' she', 'he', 'they', 'one' are used and refer to the person, object or event the writer is writing about. This narrative style is the most commonly used. Writing in the third person allows a writer to be more objective and points of view can be supported by evidence. However, direct quotes are often written in the first person.

Research and tenses
Tenses tell the reader when an event occurred in time. So, the past tense is used to express past events or completed work, present tense is used to express anything that is happening now, at this time, and future tense is used to express events that will happen in the future. When you are writing a research proposal you will always write in the future tense as you are planning research to be undertaken in the future. When writing a research paper you will usually write in the past tense. You will describe and discuss evidence gathered from literature searching and citations as well as your own research data in the past tense as these are completed tasks.

Writing preparation

Plan your paper, write an outline, think about what the focus of the paper is going to be and what sources of literature you are going to use to support your ideas or demonstrate that you have background knowledge and up-to-date information that is written on the chosen subject. You will have to be able to recognise what is **common knowledge** and in the **public domain** (no copyright restrictions), that does not need to be supported by citations, and what work needs to be acknowledged. Remember to consider the issue of plagiarism and how to avoid this by acknowledging sources of information and tools you may use. The internet is a wonderful source of information and huge volumes of data can be downloaded within minutes but you need to remember to cite internet sources and when you accessed them.

Plagiarism

What is plagiarism? Basically, it is an act of fraud and occurs when a person uses someone else's work or intellectual property without acknowledging the source or being granted permission to do so. All sources of evidence including statements and quotes need to be referenced in your writing; any validated methods or data collection tools need to be cited and some may need copyright permission. Whether writing your dissertation or a paper you have to ensure that it is your own work and that you always acknowledge the work of others.

There are computer software programmes such as Turnitin, that can be used by universities and journal editors to detect textual plagiarism. See http://www.plagiarism.org/ and http://www.turnitin.com/static/index.html for further information.

Getting your work published

Many midwives and students lack confidence to write articles. Ideally, start with an editorial or a commentary piece, then think about a short article or a discussion paper. These types of articles are referred to as opinion-based and will give readers some 'food for thought'. Focus on an issue in clinical practice or some recent event that has interested you and that you would like to share with other colleagues. If you have been involved in any new initiative or ways of working, think about writing how this came about, who was involved, how it was achieved and evaluated, and any future plans.

When writing a research paper, firstly think about how you have set out your dissertation or thesis chapters. Writing a research paper is structured very similarly. Most journals follow a similar layout and, basically, require the following sections:

- an abstract;
- short introduction;
- background;

- methodology;
- findings/results;
- discussion/limitations, conclusions;
- implications for midwifery practice.

Journals have their own house style and can use different referencing systems; you need to be aware that it can be time consuming, particularly if you have submitted to one journal, had your paper rejected and then want to submit to another journal as you will have to amend your article to fit with the second journal's house style. Having a paper rejected can be disappointing but read and consider the peer reviewers' comments, to see how you can improve and address the reasons why it was rejected. It may be that it did not fit in with the journal's specific focus or there were misunderstandings in how the paper was interpreted. Often, a paper that is submitted will need some form of revising (which can be minor or major) or further clarifications and you will be asked to amend your paper before it is considered for publication. Don't get disheartened: look upon this as a way of improving your writing skills. When you have addressed the amendments, write a covering letter to the editor and systematically list the amendments or clarifications requested and how you have addressed each of these separately. There is always some element of negotiation that can be agreed and editors can make a final decision.

It is not uncommon for peer reviewers to give some feedback that is similar and helpful, but sometimes there can be contrasting and contradicting feedback as there is always an element of subjectivity when peer reviewing papers. This is one reason that a journal will ask for at least two independent views and sometimes a third one may be requested.

Instructions for writing a paper

Articles need to be structured, using subheadings and link sentences so the article flows. All journals have guidelines on how to write a paper for their journal and are usually typewritten in their editions and on-line to help you (Box 7.3). Read them carefully and refer back to them as you are writing. Examples of the preferred referencing system are included and always check this out as there are variations. There is always guidance on word limits, depending on the type of article. More practice will improve your writing skills.

Publication bias

There appears to be an inherent bias when trying to get research published. Research that demonstrates statistically significant results has a tendency to be published and the research that does not is more likely not to get published (Dickersin, 1990).

Nonetheless, there is now an acknowledgement that research which does not demonstrate any significant results needs to be published to prevent

Box 7.3 Evidence Based Midwifery: guidelines for authors. Reproduced with permission from the Royal College of Midwives.

Aim and focus

Evidence Based Midwifery aims to promote the dissemination, implementation and evaluation of midwifery evidence at local, national and international levels. Papers on qualitative research, quantitative research, philosophical research, action research, systematic reviews and meta-analyses of qualitative or quantitative data are welcome. All authors are encouraged to discuss their research paper with peers or editorial staff with regard to issues of importance to the local, national and international readership.

The journal is published four times a year and all papers should be sent to maura@redactive.co.uk in Word for Windows format. Any hard copy material should be posted to: Maura O'Malley, Deputy Editor, *Evidence Based Midwifery*, Redactive Media Group, 17-18 Britton Street, EC1M 5TP.

Referees and review

All suitable papers submitted to *Evidence Based Midwifery* are subject to double-blinded peer review to assess their academic rigour, quality and relevance to the overall aim of the journal. Referees with relevant expertise in the subject area and/or methodology will be asked to provide a structured critical review of papers and reviews will be forwarded to the authors along with comments from the editors. Where necessary, papers will also be sent to members of the advisory panel for expert opinion on matters to do with, for example, statistical accuracy, professional relevance or legal ramifications.

All authors will receive acknowledgement of receipt of their paper and the review process should be complete within 12 weeks. Major changes will be agreed with the authors, but the editors reserve the right to make modifications in accordance with house style and demands for space and layout. All papers are sent to the first named author for essential corrections only before publication and should be returned promptly. Corrections at this proofreading stage should be kept to a minimum and references and quotations should be checked carefully. Galley proofs will be sent to all authors for final proofing prior to publication and the accuracy of the content is the responsibility of the corresponding (first) author. Figures and tables that have to be redrawn in-house may not be included with proofs. The editors will decide on the time of publication.

Authorship

(Adapted from International Committee of Medical Journal Editors, 1997)

Continued

All persons designated as authors should qualify for authorship, and all those who qualify should be listed. Each author should have participated sufficiently in the work to take public responsibility for appropriate portions of the content. One or more authors should take responsibility for the integrity of the work as a whole, from inception to published article. Authorship credit should be based only on: 1) substantial contributions to conception and design, or acquisition of data, or analysis and interpretation of data; 2) drafting the article or revising it critically for important intellectual content; and 3) final approval of the version to be published. All three conditions must be met. Acquisition of funding, the collection of data, or general supervision of the research group, by themselves, do not justify authorship. All others who contributed to the work who are not authors should be named in the acknowledgments, and what they did should be described. Increasingly, authorship of multi-centre trials is attributed to a group. All members of the group who are named as authors should fully meet the above criteria for authorship. Group members who do not meet these criteria should be listed, with their permission, in the acknowledgments or in an appendix. The order of authorship on the byline should be a joint decision of the co-authors. Authors should be prepared to explain the order in which authors are listed.

All contributors who do not meet the criteria for authorship, such as a person who provided purely technical help, writing assistance, or a department chair who provided only general support, should be listed. Financial and material support should also be acknowledged. Groups of persons who have contributed materially to the paper, but whose contributions do not justify authorship may be identified as 'clinical investigators' or 'participating investigators', and their function or contribution should be described – for example, 'served as scientific advisors', 'critically reviewed the study proposal', 'collected data', or 'provided and cared for study patients'. Because readers may infer their endorsement of the data and conclusions, all persons must have given written permission to be acknowledged.

Copyright
Evidence Based Midwifery cannot consider papers that are not original or have been submitted elsewhere, and the exclusive right to the manuscript should be set out in an accompanying statement. The author(s) transfer(s) the copyright of her or their paper to the RCM, effective if and when the paper is accepted for publication. A copyright form will be sent to each author prior to this. The copyright covers the exclusive and unlimited rights to reproduce and distribute the paper in any form of reproduction. All manuscripts should conform to the *Uniform requirements for manuscripts submitted to biomedical journals* (International Committee of Medical Journal Editors, 1997).

Style and format
Papers should be typed using double spacing with a 12pt size common font, such as 'Times' or 'Arial'. No identifying details of the authors or their institutions should appear in the submitted paper. Author details should be communicated separately, including an address to which all correspondence should be sent and a daytime telephone number. A fax number should also be included, if possible. The paper should be preceded by a structured abstract of up to 300 words that summarises the paper content. If appropriate, a suitable example would include: aim; objective; method; findings/results; and implications. The abstract should be followed by up to ten key words that identify accurately the paper's subject, purpose and focus. These key words will be used to assist indexers in cross-indexing the article and may be published with the abstract. Where approval for reproduction or modification of material is required, the principal author must obtain this. Details of sources of research funding, commercial affiliations and acknowledgements must also be included. Tables should be typed, double spaced, on separate sheets, with a short descriptive title. All relevant statistical data should be included. Illustrations are welcomed and encouraged where appropriate. Black and white photographs or transparencies are suitable. If charts or graphs are to be included, original or coordinate values should also be sent. Charts and graphs must be clearly labelled, and the axes on graphs made clear. Captions should be supplied for all illustrations. If using or adapting illustrations from another source, it is the author's responsibility to obtain written permission to reproduce the material and to credit it accordingly. All illustrations are submitted at the owner's risk. While every effort will be made to return all illustrations, the publisher accepts no liability for loss or damage while in possession of the material. Always include a citation in the text for each figure and table.

References
All work referred to in the manuscript should be fully cited using the Harvard system of referencing. The reference list should be in alphabetical and chronological order using the first author's name. All references cited must have been previously published or publicly accessible. All references in the text should be cited from primary sources and should include the authors' names and date of publication in date order. Where there are three or more authors, the first author's name followed by 'et al' is acceptable in the text, e.g. (Smith et al, 2002), but all authors must be cited in the reference list. Page numbers should be included in the text for all quotations, e.g. (Jones, 2002: 45). Reference to a journal article should include the author's surname and initials, date of publication, title of the paper, name

Continued

of the journal, volume and issue number and its first and last page numbers, e.g. Symon A. (2003) Including men in antenatal education: evaluating innovative practice. *Evidence Based Midwifery* **1(1)**: 12–19. Reference to a book should include the author, date of publication, title, publisher and town of publication, e.g. Smith A, Jones B. (1989) *Evidence Based Medicine*. BMJ Publishing Group: London. Chapters in edited books should include the additional detail of chapter title, e.g. Brown C. (1993) *Best practice*: In: Smith A, Jones B. (Eds.). *Evidence-Based Health Care*. Elsevier Science: The Netherlands.

Publication
On publication, ten print editions of the journal will be supplied to the corresponding authors of each paper, as will an electronic version.

References
International Committee of Medical Journal Editors (1997) Uniform requirements for manuscripts submitted to biomedical journals. *Annals of Internal Medicine* **126(1)**: 36–47.
Sinclair M, Ratnaike D. (2007) Writing for Evidence Based Midwifery. *Evidence Based Midwifery* **5(2)**: 66–70.

repetition and unnecessary research being undertaken. It is an ethical issue and involving service users has to be considered.

Impact of publications

It is important to publish your work and there are key journals available for midwives and student midwives to consider. See the Useful resources section later in this chapter. Some of these journals will have an impact factor (IF) value and some will not. The impact factor measures the average number of citations published in journals.

Citation data from a database produced by the Institution for Scientific Information (ISI), now part of Thomson Reuters, continuously record citations represented by the reference lists in articles for a large number of journals. The results are published as Science Citation Index (SCI).

Impact factors have a huge, but controversial, influence on the way published research is perceived and evaluated. Journals with higher impact factors are deemed to be more important than those with lower ones. A substantial number of journals are not indexed and have no impact factor. Therefore, this impact indicator is not representative of the quality of published research and there is an English language publication bias. Criticisms have been voiced on the benefits of an impact factor and there is an on-going debate on the usefulness of citation metrics. Concerns over the validity, manipulation and misuse of an impact factor have been raised (Seglen, 1997). The European

Association of Science Editors (EASE) (2008) has recently recommended that impact factors should be cautiously used for measuring and comparing journals, not used for the assessment of single papers and definitely not used for the assessment of researchers or research programmes.

This leads to the question, is the impact of an article increased by publication in an impact factor indexed journal? The answer is not necessarily and the impact needs to relate to the influence it will have on clinical practice. It is interesting to note the different impact of three midwifery research articles:

- Downe *et al.* (2001) Labour interventions associated with normal birth. In *British Journal of Midwifery* (not SCI indexed);
- Downe *et al.* (2004) A prospective randomised trial on the effect of position in the passive second-stage of labour on birth outcome in nulliparous women using epidural. In *Midwifery* (SCI indexed);
- El-Nemer *et al.* (2005) She would help me from the heart: an ethnography of Egyptian women in labour. In *Social Science & Medicine* (SCI indexed).

The *British Journal of Midwifery* article has been the most often cited, even though it is the only one without an impact factor, possibly because it caught the mood of the times, is easily accessible and it was the catalyst for the RCM Normal Birth Campaign. The *Social Science & Medicine* article is one cited by researchers in the Middle East, so it is having a different kind of impact. The *Midwifery* article is one that has been cited in the NICE intrapartum guidelines.

Publishing your work will have an impact on the knowledge base of midwifery and can influence further research and clinical practice. An example of this is research undertaken by one of the authors who has published several papers relating to localised cooling treatments to alleviate perineal trauma following childbirth. (Steen & Cooper, 1997, 1998, 1999; Steen, 2002, 2005; Steen *et al.*, 2000, 2006; Steen & Marchant, 2007). These publications have been the catalyst for midwife researchers in Mashhad, Iran to undertake a randomised controlled trial to investigate further the effectiveness of localised cooling treatments to alleviate perineal trauma (Navviba *et al.*, 2009).

Midwifery research is evolving and more and more research studies are being published. The internet has had a huge impact on how research findings and evidence are disseminated. The two examples of research undertaken in the Middle East demonstrate how it is now possible to collaborate with midwives throughout the world, regardless of language barriers, to undertake midwifery-led research.

Presenting a conference paper

Standing in front of an audience and giving an oral presentation can be a very daunting experience for many midwives and students and it is one of the reasons why you will have opportunities to do this whilst studying at both undergraduate and postgraduate level. Even experienced presenters still get nervous and have to remember to breathe and speak slowly at the commencement of the presentation, project their voice, coordinate some form of visual aid (usually PowerPoint or media) and then let the presentation flow. The more you present, the more confidence you will gain and, even though you can be nervous, you will feel a sense of achievement. You may be professionally challenged but think of this as a good thing, try not to take it personally and acknowledge your peers' views and create some discussion and debate on the subject. Remember it is so important to disseminate research and make opportunities to do so.

An example: Postures and positions in labour: best practice (Steen & Anker, 2008). See weblink: http://www.nmc-uk.org/aDisplayDocument.aspx ?documentID=5130

http://chesterrep.openrepository.com/cdr/handle/10034/48456

Useful resources

Key journals for midwives and student midwives (available on-line):
American Journal of Obstetrics and Gynecology (AJOG)
Association for Improvements in the Maternity Services (AIMS)
Birth: Issues in Perinatal Care
Birth Spiritual Journal
British Journal of Midwifery (BJM)
British Journal of Obstetrics and Gynaecology (BJOG)
British Medical Journal (BMJ)
Complementary Therapies in Nursing and Midwifery
Contraception
Disability, Pregnancy and Parenthood
Evidence Based Midwifery Journal (EBM)
Health Promotion International
International Journal of Childbirth (Note: this new journal will be on-line mid
    October 2010, hard copy January 2011)
International Journal of Gynecology and Obstetrics
Journal of Obstetrics, Gynaecology and Neonatal Nursing
Journal of Maternal and Child Health (became Family Medicine)
Journal of Nurse-Midwifery and Women Health (ACM)
Maternal and Child Health
Maternal and Child Nutrition
Maternity Matters (ARM) Journal)
Midwifery (International)
Midwifery Today
Professional Care of Mother and Child
Public Health
RCM's Midwives Journal (now Midwives Magazine and on-line papers)
Reproductive Health Matters

The African Journal of Midwifery (AJM)
The Australian Journal of Midwifery
The Journal of the American Medical Association (JAMA)
The New Zealand College of Midwives (NZCOM) Journal
The Practising Midwife
Women's Health Issues

Research networks

- Doctoral Midwifery Research Society (DMRS). See http://www.doctoralmidwiferysociety.org/default.aspx.
- A Midwifery Research List (to join). See http://www.jiscmail.ac.uk/lists/midwifery-research.html.
- A RCM Midwifery Research Group. See http://www.rcm.org.uk/college/resources/midwifery-research/.
- Internet for Midwifery. This is a free online service to help students develop their internet research skills. See http://www.vts.intute.ac.uk/tutorial/midwifery/.

Student midwifery network

SMNET: Student Midwife.NET. This is a free online service that provides student midwives with online support, educational information and an opportunity to participate in discussion and debate. See: http://www.studentmidwife.net/.

Becoming a researcher

Many midwives and student midwives are put off from undertaking research as they find it a dry subject and get confused with some of the methodologies, tools and analysis required to answer a research question.

> Midwives are so often scared off by the term research – remembering dry lectures in the classroom that involved complicated words and statistical measures that were not remotely related to them.
>
> Crozier & Macdonald, 2009.

Research is a subject in its own right and knowledge and skills take time to develop, but, with persistence, midwives and student midwives are very capable of doing this. The authors would like you to reflect on the book chapters and write something about how the book has assisted your learning and development needs, firstly on understanding research itself and, secondly, on how to undertake research. When you have achieved a better knowledge of research and successfully undertaken a research study these experiences may inspire you to want to undertake further research activities and some of you may want to become a researcher. You will certainly have gained a greater awareness and understanding of what research is, how to search and critique the evidence, what research approaches and methodologies are available and the importance of ethics and research governance.

Hicks (1996, p. 4) wrote '... *midwifery must have its own body of professional knowledge, developed by midwives for midwives, to be used by midwives. Therefore, it is imperative that a prevailing research culture is fostered within the profession.*'

Research is an essential component of midwifery and midwives must take ownership of how their profession will evolve further. Midwifery care can be enhanced by knowledge that is developed and implemented by midwives. Some research will be midwifery-led but there is also a need to undertake collaborative work with other professionals and be part of a research team.

The authors hope that some of you will be inspired to go on to do some research or further research studies that address some of the gaps in our knowledge and understanding of midwifery.

The authors would like to quote Warmel's (1996, p. 65) encouraging statement:

> In order to implement change, midwives will need to take control of their own learning process and carry out their own midwifery-led research.

For this to be achieved some midwives will need to develop and become researchers so that the theory–practice gap can be narrowed and for the profession to evolve further. It has to be recognised, however, that investment must be made in support, time and resources to do this. There are certainly barriers and challenges to overcome, but with a positive attitude and knowledge of the available evidence, changes in clinical practice that improve care and services for women, their babies and families can happen. Research evidence, writing guidelines and implementing changes in clinical practice takes time but we have to be persistent and forward thinking. A calm, confident, conscientious midwifery researcher can make a difference and have a ripple effect on many others. Midwifery researchers can take a leading role in how education, guidelines and policies inform and manage best practice. Researchers become mentors and supervise other midwives and students to become researchers; knowledge and skills to understand and undertake research are passed on.

Summary

This final chapter has focused on how to disseminate research. It has highlighted how important it is to disseminate research findings regardless of whether the results are positive or not. Guidance on writing skills and how to write a research proposal is covered in detail. A specific section on the research dissertation which covers how to plan, prepare, structure and the importance of supervision is described and discussed to helpful midwives and students undertake this task. Undertaking a dissertation is not an easy task, there is a lot to learn in a short space of time. It is a major opportunity for midwives and students to study and learn independently. It tests their ability to self-educate and enables them to take responsibility for a substantial piece of work. However, it is still important to access guidance and support to enhance the likelihood of successfully completing this task and this is stressed.

In addition, this chapter has aimed to inspire midwives and students who have undertaken a research study to write a research paper and get it published in a midwifery-related journal. How to do this and some useful advice to help a midwife or student succeed has been covered in this chapter. Presenting a conference paper is also a useful way to disseminate your work and how to do this task is also included.

It is envisaged that after reading this book some midwives and students will be inspired to continue and develop further research knowledge and skills. It is hoped that some midwives will be actively involved or undertake further research studies and some will become researchers. Some useful resources and information on becoming a researcher bring *The Handbook of Midwifery Research* to a close.

The chapters in this book have systematically covered research elements to demonstrate that is a subject in its own right. The content of this book is a stepping stone to understanding and undertaking midwifery research. The authors recommend further reading of books that specifically focus on different aspects of the research content included in this book.

Appendix A

A study exploring the relationship between midwives' attitudes to breastfeeding and their own personal experience of breastfeeding, professional experience and professional breastfeeding education.

Self completion questionnaire

Instructions:
The following questionnaire consists of four sections. Each section contains short questions. Instructions for completion are given at the beginning of each section. Most questions require only a tick in a box.

Some questions ask you to elaborate on particular aspects to find out your views and your comments to these questions will enhance the quality of the results.

The whole questionnaire should take no more than 15 to 20 minutes to complete.

Once completed please place the questionnaire, in the envelope provided, into one of the boxes in the maternity unit.

Boxes for collection of the questionnaires will be placed on Delivery Suite, postnatal and antenatal wards and also antenatal clinic.

Thank you for your participation in this study.

The Handbook of Midwifery Research, First Edition. Mary Steen and Taniya Roberts.
© 2011 Mary Steen and Taniya Roberts. Published 2011 by Blackwell Publishing Ltd.

Questionnaire

Section 1: Your current midwifery practice

Please put your answer in the space provided:

1. **Please could you state your age:**

   _____

2. **Please could you state how many years have you been working as a midwife:**

   _____

3. **Please indicate, by putting a cross in the appropriate box, your main area of current practice:**
   Community   ☐
   Hospital   ☐
   Integrated: hospital and community   ☐
   Management   ☐
   Education   ☐
   Other: please specify:

   _____

   _____

Section 2: Breastfeeding education

Please put a cross in the appropriate box and if necessary elaborate in the space provided at the end of each question.

4. **What type of education session did you received on infant feeding during your initial midwifery training?**
   One half day session   ☐
   One day   ☐
   Two days   ☐
   Module (for example 15 or 30 weeks)   ☐
   Other: please specify:

   _____

   _____

5. **What type of education session have you received on infant feeding since qualification?**
   One half day session per year ☐
   One day per year ☐
   Two days per year ☐
   Module (for example 15 or 30 weeks) ☐
   Other: please specify:

   _____

   _____

Section 3: Statements about breastfeeding

6. **For each of the following 17 statements please could you indicate, by circling the appropriate number, whether you:**
   1. strongly disagree with the statement
   2. disagree with the statement
   3. are uncertain about a response to the statement
   4. agree with the statement
   5. strongly agree with the statement

i)   The nutritional benefits of breast milk last only until the baby is weaned from breast milk
1. Strongly disagree   2. Disagree   3. Neutral   4. Agree   5. Strongly Agree

ii)   Formula feeding is more convenient than breastfeeding
1. Strongly disagree   2. Disagree   3. Neutral   4. Agree   5. Strongly Agree

iii)   Breastfeeding increases mother-infant bonding
1. Strongly disagree   2. Disagree   3. Neutral   4. Agree   5. Strongly Agree

iv)   Breast milk is lacking in iron
1. Strongly disagree   2. Disagree   3. Neutral   4. Agree   5. Strongly Agree

v)   Formula-fed babies are more likely to be overfed than breast-fed babies
1. Strongly disagree   2. Disagree   3. Neutral   4. Agree   5. Strongly Agree

Question 6: The Iowa Infant Feeding Attitude Scale (De La More, A., Russell, D.W., Dungy, C.I., Losch, M., Dusdeiker, L. (1999). The Iowa Infant Feeding Attitude Scale: Analysis of Reliability and Validity. *Journal of Applied Social Psychology.* 29, 11, 2362–2380).

vi)   Formula feeding is the better choice if a mother plans to work outside the home
1. Strongly disagree   2. Disagree   3. Neutral   4. Agree   5. Strongly Agree

vii)   Mothers who formula feed miss one of the great joys of motherhood
1. Strongly disagree   2. Disagree   3. Neutral   4. Agree   5. Strongly Agree

viii)   Women should not breastfeed in public places such as restaurants
1. Strongly disagree   2. Disagree   3. Neutral   4. Agree   5. Strongly Agree

ix)   Babies fed breast milk are healthier than babies who are fed formula
1. Strongly disagree   2. Disagree   3. Neutral   4. Agree   5. Strongly Agree

x)   Breast-fed babies are more likely to be overfed than formula-fed babies
1. Strongly disagree   2. Disagree   3. Neutral   4. Agree   5. Strongly Agree

xi)   Fathers feel left out if a mother breastfeeds
1. Strongly disagree   2. Disagree   3. Neutral   4. Agree   5. Strongly Agree

xii)   Breast milk is the ideal food for babies
1. Strongly disagree   2. Disagree   3. Neutral   4. Agree   5. Strongly Agree

xiii)   Breast milk is more easily digested than formula
1. Strongly disagree   2. Disagree   3. Neutral   4. Agree   5. Strongly Agree

xiv)   Formula is as healthy for an infant as breast milk
1. Strongly disagree   2. Disagree   3. Neutral   4. Agree   5. Strongly Agree

xv)   Breastfeeding is more convenient than formula feeding
1. Strongly disagree   2. Disagree   3. Neutral   4. Agree   5. Strongly Agree

xvi)   Breast milk is less expensive than formula
1. Strongly disagree   2. Disagree   3. Neutral   4. Agree   5. Strongly Agree

xvii)   A mother who occasionally drinks alcohol should not breastfeed her baby
1. Strongly disagree   2. Disagree   3. Neutral   4. Agree   5. Strongly Agree

Section 4: Your own breastfeeding experience
Please put a cross in the appropriate box and please could you elaborate on your answers where indicated.

7. **Have you ever breastfed a baby?**
   Yes ☐   No ☐

8. **If no, or you have not yet had children, which option would you prefer?**
   Breast ☐   Formula ☐

9. **Please could you elaborate on the reasons for your choice of response for questions 7 and 8**

   _____

   _____

   _____

   _____

   _____

   If no to question 7, please go to question 14 to add any further comments you wish in the space provided and thank you for your responses.

10. **If yes to question 7, please indicate for how long:**
    Less than 1 week   ☐
    1–2 weeks   ☐
    3–4 weeks   ☐
    5–8 weeks   ☐
    9–12 weeks   ☐
    3–6 months   ☐
    More than 6 months   ☐

11. **If yes to question 7, did you find the experience:**
    Positive ☐   Negative ☐   Negative and positive ☐

12. **Please could you elaborate on your reasons for your response to question 11:**

    _____

    _____

    _____

    _____

    _____

13. **If you had another baby would you breastfeed?**
    Yes ☐   No ☐

14. **Please add any further comments you wish:**

_____

_____

_____

_____

_____

_____

_____

Thank you for taking time to complete this questionnaire.

Appendix B

Covering letter

Dear _____

Re: Midwifery research study

Do specific antenatal sessions influence how you choose to deliver your baby if you have already had a Caesarean section?

Hello,

My name is _____ and I am a midwife at _____.

I am going to undertake research into the possible impact specific antenatal sessions have on how women choose to deliver their baby following a previous Caesarean section. After a Caesarean section, the majority of women have the option to choose either a vaginal birth after Caesarean (VBAC) or an elective repeat Caesarean section (ERCS) in a subsequent pregnancy.

It has been identified that you have already had a Caesarean section and that you are a suitable candidate to be invited to consent to participating in the study.

Permission has been granted from the _____ ethics committee, the _____ regional ethics committee and the Research and Development department at _____ and your Obstetric Consultant to invite you to participate in a study. The study will explore the effect of specific antenatal sessions on your decision for mode of delivery during this pregnancy.

Further information relating to this research study is written in the participation information leaflet.

Many thanks for taking the time to read this letter.

Signed

Midwife/researcher

The Handbook of Midwifery Research, First Edition. Mary Steen and Taniya Roberts.
© 2011 Mary Steen and Taniya Roberts. Published 2011 by Blackwell Publishing Ltd.

Appendix C

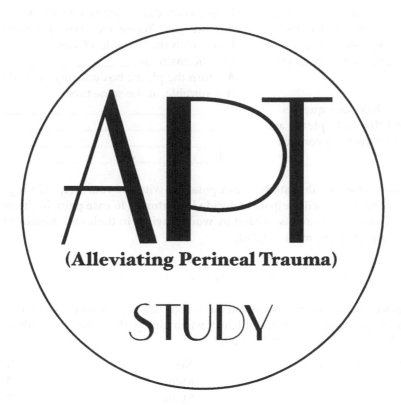

(Alleviating Perineal Trauma)

STUDY

Mother's questionnaire

Trial Number:

Group: _____

Congratulations on the birth of your baby

Please take a few minutes to complete this questionnaire during the first 5 days following the birth of your baby, then at 10 days and finally at 14 days. We would also like to follow up at 3 months. We are really interested in how you are feeling and the pain you may have felt (around the area where your stitches are) during this period of time. We are also interested in your views concerning the availability and effectiveness of treatments when in hospital and when in your own home.

Home Visits

Please ask the community midwife to complete the Green Questionnaire in your folder when she visits you.

If you have any queries about the study please ask your midwife or contact:

At the end of the trial

Please ask the community midwife to:
♦ return your Yellow Questionnaire in the folder with the midwife's Green Questionnaire to _____
♦ return the plastic box and any gel pads, if applicable, at the same time.

_____
_____
_____
Tel _____ or _____

Please remember this study is not possible without your help. Giving us this information will help us to decide if treatment to ease pain, in the area where the stitches are, is needed by women when in their own homes and, if so, which is the most helpful.

Day 1 – Please answer these questions, it should only take about 5 minutes.

1. Since your delivery, how much pain have you experienced from the area around where you were stitched when doing the following activities: (*Please tick one box for each activity*):

Walking about	None	❐
	Mild	❐
	Moderate	❐
	Severe	❐
Sitting down	None	❐
	Mild	❐
	Moderate	❐
	Severe	❐
Lying in bed	None	❐
	Mild	❐
	Moderate	❐
	Severe	❐

2. What words would you use to describe the pain you have felt in the last 24 hours:

_____

_____

_____

3. Since your delivery, have you experienced pain from haemorrhoids (piles)?
Yes ☐
No ☐
Unsure ☐

If Yes, would you describe your pain as:
None ☐
Mild ☐
Moderate ☐
Severe ☐

4. Since your delivery, please name the tablets and how many you have taken to relieve the pain felt from around where the stitches are:

_____

_____

Please name any other treatment used to relieve the pain:

_____

_____

5. **If applicable**, in the last 24 hours, how many cold treatments have you applied to the area where the stitches are?

If not applicable, please go to question 12.

6. During use of the cooling device is the pain:
Worse ☐
The same ☐
Less ☐
Stopped ☐

7. Do you think that the cooling device, when applied for the first 10 minutes, is:

Too cold ❐
Not cold enough ❐
About right ❐

8. Did you find the cooling device:

Easy to use ❐
Difficult to use ❐
Neither ❐

9. Did you find the cooling device:

Comfortable ❐
Uncomfortable ❐
Neither ❐

10. Do you think that the cooling effect is:

Too short ❐
Too long ❐
About right ❐

11. How would you rate the effectiveness of the cooling treatments you have applied?

Poor ❐
Fair ❐
Good ❐
Very good ❐
Excellent ❐

12. How are you feeding your baby?

Breast ❐
Bottle ❐
Both ❐

13. Has pain or discomfort from the area around the stitches made it difficult for you to feed your baby?

Yes ❐
No ❐

Day 2 – Please answer these questions, it should only take about 5 minutes.

14. In the last 24 hours, how much pain have you experienced from the area around where you were stitched when doing the following activities: *(Please tick one box for each activity):*

Walking about	None	❏
	Mild	❏
	Moderate	❏
	Severe	❏
Sitting down	None	❏
	Mild	❏
	Moderate	❏
	Severe	❏
Lying in bed	None	❏
	Mild	❏
	Moderate	❏
	Severe	❏

15. What words would you use to describe the pain you have felt in the last 24 hours:

_____

_____

_____

16. In the last 24 hours, have you experienced pain from haemorrhoids?

Yes	❏
No	❏
Unsure	❏

Would you describe your pain as:

None	❏
Mild	❏
Moderate	❏
Severe	❏

17. Since your delivery, please name the tablets and how many you have taken to relieve the pain felt from around where the stitches are:

_____

_____

Please name any other treatment used to relieve the pain:

_____

_____

18. **If applicable**, in the last 24 hours, how many cold treatments have you applied to the area where the stitches are?

☐

If not applicable, please go to question 25.

19. During use of the cooling device is the pain:
Worse ☐
The same ☐
Less ☐
Stopped ☐

20. Do you think that the cooling device, when applied for the first 10 minutes, is:
Too cold ☐
Not cold enough ☐
About right ☐

21. Did you find the cooling device:
Easy to use ☐
Difficult to use ☐
Neither ☐

22. Did you find the cooling device:
Comfortable ☐
Uncomfortable ☐
Neither ☐

23. Do you think that the cooling effect is:
Too short ☐
Too long ☐
About right ☐

24. How would you rate the effectiveness of the cooling treatments you have applied?
Poor ☐
Fair ☐
Good ☐
Very good ☐
Excellent ☐

25. How are you feeding your baby?
Breast   ❐
Bottle   ❐
Both   ❐

26. Has pain or discomfort from the area around the stitches made it difficult for you to feed your baby?
Yes   ❐
No   ❐

Day 3 – Please answer these questions, it should only take about 5 minutes.

27. In the last 24 hours, how much pain have you experienced from the area around where you were stitched when doing the following activities: *(Please tick one box for each activity):*

Walking about	None	❐
	Mild	❐
	Moderate	❐
	Severe	❐
Sitting down	None	❐
	Mild	❐
	Moderate	❐
	Severe	❐
Lying in bed	None	❐
	Mild	❐
	Moderate	❐
	Severe	❐

28. What words would you use to describe the pain you have felt in the last 24 hours:

_____

_____

_____

29. In the last 24 hours, have you experienced pain from haemorrhoids?
Yes   ❐
No   ❐
Unsure   ❐

Would you describe your pain as:
None   ❐
Mild   ❐
Moderate   ❐
Severe   ❐

30. Since your delivery, please name the tablets and how many you have taken to relieve the pain felt from around where the stitches are:

_____

_____

Please name any other treatment used to relieve the pain:

_____

_____

31. **If applicable**, in the last 24 hours, how many cold treatments have you applied to the area where the stitches are?

☐

If not applicable, please go to question 38.

32. During use of the cooling device is the pain:
Worse ☐
The same ☐
Less ☐
Stopped ☐

33. Do you think that the cooling device, when applied for the first 10 minutes, is:
Too cold ☐
Not cold enough ☐
About right ☐

34. Did you find the cooling device:
Easy to use ☐
Difficult to use ☐
Neither ☐

35. Did you find the cooling device:
Comfortable ☐
Uncomfortable ☐
Neither ☐

36. Do you think that the cooling effect is:
Too short ☐
Too long ☐
About right ☐

37. How would you rate the effectiveness of the cooling treatments you have applied?

Poor ☐

Fair ☐

Good ☐

Very good ☐

Excellent ☐

38. How are you feeding your baby?

Breast ☐

Bottle ☐

Both ☐

39. Has pain or discomfort from the area around the stitches made it difficult for you to feed your baby?

Yes ☐

No ☐

Day 4 – Please answer these questions, it should only take about 5 minutes.

40. In the last 24 hours, how much pain have you experienced from the area around where you were stitched when doing the following activities: *(Please tick one box for each activity):*

Walking about	None	☐
	Mild	☐
	Moderate	☐
	Severe	☐
Sitting down	None	☐
	Mild	☐
	Moderate	☐
	Severe	☐
Lying in bed	None	☐
	Mild	☐
	Moderate	☐
	Severe	☐

41. What words would you use to describe the pain you have felt in the last 24 hours:

_____

_____

_____

42. In the last 24 hours, have you experienced pain from haemorrhoids?
Yes ☐
No ☐
Unsure ☐

Would you describe your pain as:
None ☐
Mild ☐
Moderate ☐
Severe ☐

43. Since your delivery, please name the tablets and how many you have taken to relieve the pain felt from around where the stitches are:

_____

_____

Please name any other treatment used to relieve the pain:

_____

_____

44. If applicable, in the last 24 hours, how many cold treatments have you applied to the area where the stitches are?

☐

If not applicable, please go to question 51.

45. During use of the cooling device is the pain:
Worse ☐
The same ☐
Less ☐
Stopped ☐

46. Do you think that the cooling device, when applied for the first 10 minutes, is:
Too cold ☐
Not cold enough ☐
About right ☐

47. Did you find the cooling device:
Easy to use ☐
Difficult to use ☐
Neither ☐

48. Did you find the cooling device:
    Comfortable   ❏
    Uncomfortable   ❏
    Neither   ❏

49. Do you think that the cooling effect is:
    Too short   ❏
    Too long   ❏
    About right   ❏

50. How would you rate the effectiveness of the cooling treatments you have applied?
    Poor   ❏
    Fair   ❏
    Good   ❏
    Very good   ❏
    Excellent   ❏

51. How are you feeding your baby?
    Breast   ❏
    Bottle   ❏
    Both   ❏

52. Has pain or discomfort from the area around the stitches made it difficult for you to feed your baby?
    Yes   ❏
    No   ❏

Day 5 – Please answer these questions, it should only take about 5 minutes.

53. In the last 24 hours, how much pain have you experienced from the area around where you were stitched when doing the following activities: *(Please tick one box for each activity)*:

Walking about	None	❏
	Mild	❏
	Moderate	❏
	Severe	❏
Sitting down	None	❏
	Mild	❏
	Moderate	❏
	Severe	❏
Lying in bed	None	❏
	Mild	❏
	Moderate	❏
	Severe	❏

54. What words would you use to describe the pain you have felt in the last 24 hours:

_____

_____

_____

55. In the last 24 hours, have you experienced pain from haemorrhoids?
Yes ☐
No ☐
Unsure ☐

Would you describe your pain as:
None ☐
Mild ☐
Moderate ☐
Severe ☐

56. Since your delivery, please name the tablets and how many you have taken to relieve the pain felt from around where the stitches are:

_____

_____

Please name any other treatment used to relieve the pain:

_____

_____

57. **If applicable**, in the last 24 hours, how many cold treatments have you applied to the area where the stitches are?

☐

If not applicable, please go to question 64.

58. During use of the cooling device is the pain:
Worse ☐
The same ☐
Less ☐
Stopped ☐

59. Do you think that the cooling device, when applied for the first 10 minutes, is:

Too cold ❐

Not cold enough ❐

About right ❐

60. Did you find the cooling device:

Easy to use ❐

Difficult to use ❐

Neither ❐

61. Did you find the cooling device:

Comfortable ❐

Uncomfortable ❐

Neither ❐

62. Do you think that the cooling effect is:

Too short ❐

Too long ❐

About right ❐

63. How would you rate the effectiveness of the cooling treatments you have applied?

Poor ❐

Fair ❐

Good ❐

Very good ❐

Excellent ❐

64. How are you feeding your baby?

Breast ❐

Bottle ❐

Both ❐

65. Has pain or discomfort from the area around the stitches made it difficult for you to feed your baby?

Yes ❐

No ❐

Day 10 – Please answer these questions, it should only take about 5 minutes.

66. In the last 24 hours, how much pain have you experienced from the area around where you were stitched when doing the following activities: *(Please tick one box for each activity):*

Walking about	None	❒
	Mild	❒
	Moderate	❒
	Severe	❒
Sitting down	None	❒
	Mild	❒
	Moderate	❒
	Severe	❒
Lying in bed	None	❒
	Mild	❒
	Moderate	❒
	Severe	❒

67. In the last 24 hours, have you experienced pain from haemorrhoids?

Yes	❒
No	❒
Unsure	❒

Would you describe your pain as:

None	❒
Mild	❒
Moderate	❒
Severe	❒

68. Since your delivery, please name the tablets and how many you have taken to relieve the pain felt from around where the stitches are:

_____

_____

Please name any other treatment used to relieve the pain:

_____

69. **If applicable**, over the last 5 days, have you applied any cooling treatment to the area where you were stitched?

Yes	❒
No	❒

If yes, how many times?

❒

If not applicable, please go to question 72.

70. Do you think it is important to have cooling treatments available for use in your own home?
Yes ⬜
No ⬜

How important do you think this is?
Not important ⬜
Important ⬜
Very important ⬜

71. How are you feeding your baby?
Breast ⬜
Bottle ⬜
Both ⬜

72. Has pain or discomfort from the area around the stitches made it difficult for you to feed your baby?
Yes ⬜
No ⬜

73. How would you rate your level of satisfaction with the overall care you have received for the area around where you were stitched?
Poor ⬜
Fair ⬜
Good ⬜
Very good ⬜
Excellent ⬜

Day 14 – Please answer these questions, it should only take about 5 minutes.

74. Is there anything else you would like to tell us about the treatment you have received for the area around where the stitches were?

_____

_____

_____

_____

_____

_____

_____

75. How important do you think it is for you to be involved in your own care following the birth of your baby?

Not important ☐

Important ☐

Very important ☐

76. If you have had a baby before what was your experience, if any, of pain and discomfort from stitches following the birth?

_____

_____

_____

_____

_____

_____

_____

77. Would you be willing to complete a short postal questionnaire in about 3 months' time?

Yes ☐

No ☐

Please give the midwife this completed questionnaire in the trial folder

The midwife will then return it to: _____

_____

Thank you for your help in this study.

Appendix D

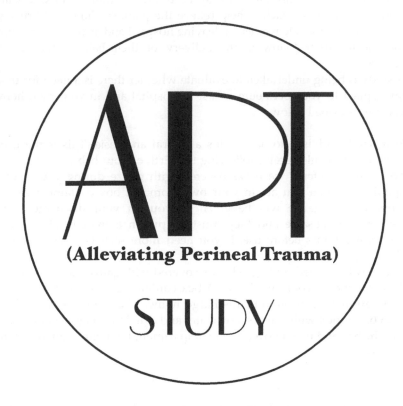

(Alleviating Perineal Trauma)
STUDY

Women's information leaflet

Midwives are always trying to improve the care you receive.
Would you like to help us with our research?

What is this study about?

Midwives are increasingly concerned with improving the care you receive both in hospital and in your own home. This requires the midwives to offer advice and support following the birth of your baby and to promote the use of self-care, especially in the home setting.

Sometimes, when your baby is being born, your perineum (the part of your body between the opening to your vagina and back passage) can tear or it may be necessary, with your consent, for a midwife to perform a cut (episiotomy). Injury to your perineum may involve stitching and, as with other forms of injury, pain, swelling and bruising may occur.

While you are in hospital you may be offered bathing, painkillers and sometimes a small ice pack to help relieve the pain, swelling and bruising. Pain relief is not given to women on leaving hospital and as women are going home much earlier following the delivery of their babies this may be necessary.

A study is being undertaken to evaluate whether there is a need for treatment applied to your perineum whilst in hospital and in your own home. These are described below:

• You will be advised to have baths and oral analgesia. This is the usual treatment you would receive following the birth of your baby.
• You may be offered ice packs covered with gauze during your stay in hospital and when you are in your own home. A box containing sachets (to freeze) and gauze will be given to you on your discharge home. These are not reusable and they must be put in a freezer compartment for at least 2 hours before use. If you need more sachets please ask your midwife.
• You may be offered cooling gel pads covered with gauze during your stay in hospital and in your own home. A box containing 3 gel pads and gauze will be given to you on your discharge home. These are reusable. These should be cleaned with warm soapy water and dried thoroughly before being put in the box and then into a freezer compartment for a minimum of 2 hours before use.

What will I have to do?

You will be asked to describe and rate the pain you have felt over the previous 24 hours on: Day 1, Day 2, Day 3, Day 4, Day 5, Day 10 and finally on Day 14, following the birth of your baby. We would also like to follow up at 3 months, if you give your consent.

What will the midwife have to do?

A midwife will examine you on these days to assess for any swelling, bruising and healing of the wound. She will also observe to see if the stitches are softening and absorbing.

Do I have to participate in this study?

If you have had a normal delivery and have had some stitches, the midwife looking after you in labour will ask if you are willing to take part in this study. If you agree you will be asked to sign a consent form.

It is your choice, you are free to withdraw at any time and this will not affect your care in any way. If you do not wish to be in the study you will be offered the usual method of treatment.

Who has given approval for this study?

This study has the approval of the _____ Research Ethics Committee and is fully supported by _____ Hospital.

Who is funding the study?

This study is funded by the _____.

Further information

If you would like further information please do not hesitate to ask your midwife or contact:

Mary Steen,
Study Co-ordinator
Tel: _____.

Abstract – a succinct, but brief (100–150 words) summary, that gives an overview of the study and its findings. It captures the readers' attention to the relevance of the article to themselves.

Action research – aims to implement and evaluate changes in practice; it is cyclical in nature. A problem is identified, change is initiated, evidence is gathered to assess the effectiveness of the change, further refinements may be required and assessments conducted until an improvement/benefit is demonstrated. Can follow both qualitative and quantitative approaches.

Aim – what is hoped will be achieved.

Analysis – systematic process of making sense of results.

Anonymity – the identity of individuals who have taken part in the study cannot be established from the collected data.

Audit trail – a process used by qualitative researchers, so that other researchers can follow the decisions and interpretations used by the researchers which adds to the credibility of the study.

Bibliography – a list of the sources of information used during the study.

Case study – in-depth study of a location (Delivery Suite) or single individual.

Citation – the source of information used.

Clinical trial – experimental research that tests the effectiveness of a clinical treatment/intervention.

Coding – the process of breaking down qualitative data by giving it a name/label/category to help establish recurring themes.

Cohort – a defined total group that is studied over time.

Confirmability – refers to the data being true representations of the information that the participants have provided (not influenced/biased by the researcher).

Convenience sampling – the researcher selects the most easily accessible people from the population.

The Handbook of Midwifery Research, First Edition. Mary Steen and Taniya Roberts.
© 2011 Mary Steen and Taniya Roberts. Published 2011 by Blackwell Publishing Ltd.

Copyright – legal protection of intellectual property and the exclusive rights to distribution, use and reproduction of the material

Correlation – a statistical procedure that searches for a relationship between two variables.

Credibility – ensures in qualitative research that the findings of a study are a true representation of participant-provided data.

Critical appraisal – refers to a balanced scrutiny of a research paper, highlighting its strengths and weaknesses and applying these judgements to practice.

Data – information collected by researchers during a study.

Data analysis – the process of examining the data to make sense of them.

Data saturation – used in qualitative research to signify when no new information is revealed, to bring data collection to an end.

Data set – all the data for a research study.

Deductive – belongs to quantitative research and means theories, propositions or hypothesis (logical reasoning) about the research outcome.

Delphi study – a process of developing ideas and forming a consensus about an issue among a group of people, who are considered to be experts on the topic without them being in contact with each other.

Dependability – refers to the stability (reliability) of data over time and conditions.

Dependent variable – the effect measured in an experimental study.

Descriptive statistics – refers to the organisation and analysis of numerical data, presented in graphs or tables.

Dissemination – the results/findings of a research study communicated to others by either publication, conference presentations, seminars or reports.

Emic – refers to researcher's point of view in ethnography.

Epistemology – the study of the nature of knowledge, how we understand our world and relate this to the understanding of theories of what makes up knowledge. It concerns questioning and understanding how we know what we know.

Ethical approval – formal approval that proposed research is ethical.

Ethnography – a research methodology that can enable researchers to make sense of people's actions by observing them in the context of their environment.

Etic – refers to participants' point of view in ethnography.

Feminist research – not just research on women conducted by women, it is much more complex than that. It is about recognising oppression and the reasons for it, valuing women's experiences and understanding the actions that can be taken to change the situation.

Field notes – written accounts made from observations.

Focus group – a research method that involves a group of people who are asked about or in some circumstances given a research problem to discuss. Each group is assigned a facilitator to aid the flow of discussion and ensure everyone has a voice.

Gantt chart – a type of bar chart that can be used to illustrate the start and finish dates and significant phases and milestones for a research project.

Generalise – apply results from a quantitative study to the population from where the sample was derived.

Grounded theory – focuses on generating a theory from research data, to describe and explain what is happening in a social setting or interaction.

Historical research – about examining events in the past that can be related to current practice.

Hypothesis – the researcher's prediction/proposition about the outcome of the study (experimental), focusing on the relationship between the independent and dependent variables.

Inclusion criteria – attributes or characteristics of potential participants that ensure they should be included in the study.

Independent variable – the intervention that is being investigated in an experimental study.

Inductive – developing or generating theory from data.

Inferential statistics – uses numerical results from an experimental study to infer that these findings can be generalised to the population.

Informed consent – individuals who are invited to take part in a study are asked their permission to participate dependent on the fact that they fully understand what is involved and that they can withdraw from the study at any time without adverse consequences.

Interval/ratio data – data that are recorded on a scale with equal distance between points.

Interview – data collection tool, which involves verbal communication with an individual or group.

Literature review – an analysis of published research on a particular topic.

Longitudinal study – follows the particular research issue over time, the data are therefore collected at intervals to determine any change.

Mean – refers to the average measurement in quantitative research.

Median – the centre value for a set of figures.

Method – comprises the procedural steps for data collection and data analysis.

Methodology – refers to the theoretical and philosophical underpinnings of the research and the knowledge that is to be determined or theory developed.

Mode – a measurement of central tendency, the most frequent value found in a set of numbers.

Narrative research – essentially the collection and analysis of stories.

Naturalistic paradigm – often considered to be an alternative paradigm to the positivist one. It maintains that there are multiple interpretations of reality and that the goal of research is to understand how individuals construct reality within their context. It is subjective and is associated with qualitative research.

Non-participant observation – the observer records observations without any interactions within the setting that is being studied.

Non-probability sampling – the chance of any individual being selected is not known.

Objectivity – the researcher remains detached from the research.

Observation – data collection tool by visual means.

Ontology – concerns our views about what constitutes the social world and how we can go about studying it, therefore ontological assumptions are the researcher's views about the nature of reality.

Open sampling – requires the researcher to be open to interviewing any participant, observing any events.

Ordinal data – categorical data which are gathered into groups e.g. age group.

Paradigm – a view, belief, school of thought which the researcher follows to guide knowledge acquisition.

Participant – a person taking part in a research study.

Participant observation – the researcher tries to become part of the culture by being in the 'field', rather than from a detached stance.

Phenomenology – the goal of phenomenological enquiry is to fully describe a lived experience. It therefore answers questions of meaning, in understanding an experience from those who have experienced it.

Pilot study – a small study to ensure that the larger study will have reliability, a test run usually used in quantitative research.

Population – all people from which data can be collected, e.g. pregnant women – a subset of this group is called the sample.

Positivist paradigm – considered to be the traditional paradigm underlying the scientific approach. This paradigm assumes that there is a fixed, orderly reality that can be objectively studied. It is associated with quantitative research.

Power calculation – a calculation which is conducted at the design stage of an experimental study, e.g. randomised controlled trial, survey, to determine the sample size required to ensure statistically significant results are achieved.

Probability sample – all the people in the target population have a known chance (more than a zero chance) of being chosen to be part of the sample.

Purposive sample – the participants are known to possess key characteristics which can best inform the research, therefore the participants are essentially selected to take part.

P-value – the probability of a result happening by chance.

Qualitative approach – involves exploring opinions, behaviours and experiences from the participants' points of view, thereby determining what something means from the perspectives of those taking part in a research study and is inductive and subjective.

Quantitative approach – centred within empirical knowledge, facts, figures, experiments, and is therefore tangible, deductive and objective.

Questionnaire – data collection tool, which encompasses a list of questions in written format.

Quota sample – a sample chosen as a cross-section of participants directly proportional to the age, gender, martial status, etc. of the population.

Random sample – a sample which gives every individual an equal chance of being chosen.

Randomised controlled trial – type of clinical trial where participants are allocated randomly to the intervention or control group and where the dependent and independent variables are analysed to assess clinical effectiveness.

Rating scale – a scale that allows participants to rate their preferences.

Raw data – data before they have been analysed.

Reflexivity – is integral to qualitative research as it involves researchers acknowledging their personal biases, therefore being self-aware.

Reliability – the accuracy and consistency of the data collection tool in quantitative research.

Research – can be depicted as systematic process, which requires a series of actions to either answer a question, verify a hunch or to test a theory, therefore generating new knowledge or refining existing information.

Research design – a detailed plan of the research study.

Research question – a specific question that guides the research process.

Sample – group/culture/organisation which represents the population.

Semi-structured interview – a type of interview used in qualitative research. The types of questions asked are usually 'open'. An open-ended question such as 'can you tell me more about...can you tell me why?' is hoping to elicit information from the participant's perspective yet it is focused on the research topic.

Snowball sample – the researcher identifies some individuals who possess the necessary characteristics/experiences and then asks these to suggest others who may be willing to participate.

Statistics – methods to analyse numerical data.

Structured interview – the same questions are asked to each participant in the same order.

Survey – a non-experimental quantitative study, which uses questionnaires or interviews to collect information from a large sample of the population.

Systematic review – all available research evidence, usually quantitative but can be qualitative, on a topic is analysed and evaluated to guide best practice.

Thematic analysis – qualitative data, that are usually gathered from interviews, are analysed for themes and meanings.

Theory – a set of ideas that guides a study.

Transferability – refers to the extent to which the study's findings can be transferred to other settings or groups.

Trustworthiness – about ensuring that qualitative research represents the truth. It encompasses credibility, transferability, dependability and confirmability.

Validity – the extent to which a data collection tool has produced what it was intended to.

References

Ahn E, Pairaudeau N, Pairaudeau N Jr, Cerat Y, Couturier B, Fortier A, Paradis E, Koren G (2006) A randomised cross over trial of tolerability and compliance of a micronutrient supplement with low iron separated from calcium vs high iron combined with calcium in pregnant women. *BMC Pregnancy and Childbirth*, doi: 10.1186/1471-2393 -6-10.

Albers LL (1999) The duration of labor in healthy women. *Journal of Perinatology* **19**(2): 114–119.

Albers LL, Schiff M, Gorwoda JG (1996) The length of active labor in normal pregnancies. *Obstetrics and Gynecology* **87**: 355–359.

Altman DG, Doré CJ (1990) Randomisation and baseline comparisons in clinical trials. *Lancet* **335**: 149–153. (PMID: 0001967441).

Altman DG, Schulz KF, Moher D, Egger M, Davidoff F, Elbourne D, Gøtzsche PC, Lang T (2001) The revised CONSORT statement for reporting randomized trials: explanation and elaboration. *Annals of Internal Medicine* **134**(8): 663–694.

Annells M (1996) Hermeneutic phenomenology: philosophical perspectives and current use in nursing research. *Journal of Advanced Nursing* **23**: 705–713.

Armstrong N (2010) Clinical mentors' influence on student midwives clinical practice. *British Journal of Midwifery* **18**(2): 114–125.

Baker L (2006) Ten common pitfalls to avoid when conducting qualitative research. *British Journal of Midwifery* **14**(9): 530–531.

Barbour R (2008) *Introducing Qualitative Research*. Sage Publications, Thousand Oaks, CA.

Barbour R, Kitzinger J (1999) *Developing Focus Group Research: Politics, Theory, and Practice*. Sage Publications, London.

Barclay L, Martin N (1983) A sensitive area: care of the episiotomy in the post-partum period. *Australian Journal of Advanced Nursing* **1**(1): 12–19.

Barnett-Page E, Thomas J (2009) *Methods for the synthesis of qualitative research: a critical review*. ERSC. Evidence for Policy and Practice Information and Co-ordinating, EPPI Centre, London. http://eppi.ioe.ac.uk/cms/Default.aspx?tabid=188. Last accessed 21/03/10.

Baxby D (1981) *Jenner's Smallbox Vaccine*, Vol 1. Heinemann Educational Books Ltd, London, 1–196.

The Handbook of Midwifery Research, First Edition. Mary Steen and Taniya Roberts.
© 2011 Mary Steen and Taniya Roberts. Published 2011 by Blackwell Publishing Ltd.

Bazanger I (1997) Deciphering chronic pain. In: A Strauss, J Corbin, eds. *Grounded Theory in Practice*. Sage Publications, Thousand Oaks, CA, 1–34.

Beauchamp T, Childress J (2001) *Principles of Biomedical Ethics*, 5th edn. Oxford University Press, Oxford.

Beck CT (1994) Phenomenology: its use in nursing research. *International Journal of Nursing Studies* **31**(6): 499–510.

Beckley S, Stenhouse E, Greene K (2000) The development and evaluation of a computer-assisted teaching programme for intrapartum fetal monitoring. *British Journal of Obstetrics & Gynaecology* **107**: 1138–1144.

Begley C (2008) Approaches to research. In: R Watson, H McKenna, S Cowman, J Keady, eds. *Nursing Research Designs and Methods*. Churchill Livingstone Elsevier, Edinburgh, 13–22.

Bell J (2005) *Doing your Research Project: A Guide for First-Time Researcher in Education*, 4th edn. Open University Press, Maidenhead.

Belmont Report (1979) *Regulations and Ethical Guidelines, Ethical Principles and Guidelines for the Protection of Human Subjects of Research*. Office of Human Subjects. http://ohsr.od.nih.gov/guidelines/belmont.html. Last accessed 9/6/10.

Berg M, Dahlberg K (1998) A phenomenological study of women's experiences of complicated childbirth. *Midwifery* **14**: 23–29.

Bland M (2003) *An Introduction to Medical Statistics*, 3rd edn. Oxford University Press, Oxford.

Blaxter L, Hughes C, Tight M (2006) *How to Research*, 3rd edn. Open Unversity Press, Maidenhead.

Bluff R (1997) Evaluating qualitative research. *British Journal of Midwifery* **5**(4): 232–324.

Bluff R (2006) Grounded theory. In: ER Cluett, R Bluff, eds. *Principles and Practice of Research in Midwifery*, 2nd edn. Elsevier, Edinburgh, 153–170.

Bowers D (2002) *Medical Statistics from Scratch*. John Wiley and Sons Ltd., Chichester.

Bowling A (2009) *Research Methods in Health: Investigating Health and Health Services*, 3rd edn. Open University Press, Maidenhead.

Boychuk Duchscher JE, Morgan D (2004) Grounded theory: reflections on the emergence vs. forcing debate. *Journal of Advanced Nursing* **48**(6): 605–612

Brett-Davies M (2007) *Doing a Successful Research Project: Using Qualitative or Quantitative Methods*. Palgrave MacMillan, New York.

Brewer JD (2000) *Ethnography*. Open University Press, Buckingham.

Brindle S, Douglas F, Van Teijlingen S, Hundley V (2005) Midwifery research: questionnaire survey. *RCM Midwives Journal* **8**(4): 156–158.

Brink PJ, Edgecombe N (2003) What is becoming of ethnography? *Qualitative Health Research* **13**(7): 1028–1030.

Bryman A (2008) *Social Research Methods*. Oxford University Press, Oxford.

Burns N, Grove SK (2009) *The Practice of Nursing Research*, 6th edn. Saunders Elsevier, St Louis, MO.

Busse R, Worz M (2003) German plans for health care modernisation. *Euro-Health* **9**(1): 21–24.

Calderdale and Huddersfield NHS Trust (2004) *Clinical Audit of Moxibustion Therapy*. Calderdale and Huddersfield NHS Trust, Calderdale, West Yorkshire.

Camacho-Sandoval J (2007) *GPower tutorial*. Heinrich-Heine-Universität: Dusseldorf. http://www.psycho.uni-duesseldorf.de/abteilungen/aap/gpower3/. Last accessed 27/3/10.

Campbell MJ, Julious SA, Altman DG (1995) Estimating sample sizes for binary, ordered categorical, and continuous outcomes in two group comparisons. *British Medical Journal* **311**: 1145–1148.

Carpenter DR (1999) Phenomenology as method. In: HJ Streubert, DR Carpenter, eds. *Qualitative Research in Nursing: Advancing the Humanistic Imperative*, 2nd edn. Lippincott, Philadelphia, PA, 43–63.

Carpenter DR (2007) Phenomenology as method. In: HJS Speziale, DR Carpenter, eds. *Qualitative Research in Nursing: Advancing the Humanistic Imperative*, 4th edn. Lippincott, Williams & Wilkins, Philadelphia, PA, 75–102.

Carter B (2004) How do you analyse qualitative data? In: T Lavender, G Edwards, Z Alfirevic, eds. *Demystifying Qualitative Research in Pregnancy and Childbirth*. Quay Books, Salisbury, 87–107.

Carthey J (2003) The role of structured observational research in health care. *Quality & Safety in Health Care* **12**(Supp 2): ii13–ii16.

Cartwright A (1986) *Health Surveys in Practice and Potential*, 2nd edn. King Edward's Hospital Fund for London, London.

Casey D, Devane D (2010) Midwifery basics: understanding research (3). Sampling. *Practising Midwife* **13**(1): 40–43.

Chalmers I, Enkin M, Keirse MJNC (1989) *Effective Care in Pregnancy and Childbirth*, Vol 1 and II. Oxford University Press, Oxford.

Charmaz K (2006) *Constructing Grounded Theory*. Sage Publications, London.

Clapp JF (2000) Exercise during pregnancy. A clinical update. *Clinics in Sports Medicine* **2**: 273–286.

Clark E (2000) The historical context of research in midwifery. In: S Proctor, M Renfrew, eds. *Linking Research & Practice in Midwifery*. Bailliere Tindall, London, 35–54.

Clemmens D (2003) Adolescent motherhood: a meta-synthesis of qualitative studies. *American Journal of Maternal and Child Nursing* **28**: 23–29.

Cluett ER, Bluff R (2006) *Principles and Practice of Research in Midwifery*, 2nd edn. Churchill Livingstone, Edinburgh.

CMACE-RCOG (2010) *Management of Women with Obesity in Pregnancy*. Centre for Maternal and Child Enquires and Royal College of Obstetricians and Gynaecologists, London. http://www.cmace.org.uk/getdoc/1812417f-de48-4291-a58c-e85b87bc95fc/CMACE-RCOG-Joint-Guideline_Management-of-Women-wi.aspx. Last accessed 25/03/10.

Cohen J (1960) A co-efficient of agreement for nominal scales. *Educational & Psychological Measurement* **20**: 37–46.

Cohen MZ (2000) Introduction. In: MZ Cohen, DL Kahn, RH Steeves, eds. *Hermeutic Pheneomenlogical Research: a Practical Guide for Nurse Researchers*. Sage Publications, Thousand Oaks, CA.

Cohen MZ (2002) Introduction to qualitative research. In: G LoBiondo-Wood, J Haber, eds. *Nursing Research Methods, Critical Appraisal & Utilisation*, 5th edn. Mosby, St Louis, MO, 125–138.

Cohen MZ, Kahn DL, Steeves RH (2000) *Hermeutic Pheneomenlogical Research: a Practical Guide for Nurse Researchers*. Sage Publications, Thousand Oaks, CA.

Colaizzi PF (1978) Psychological research as the phenomenologist views it. In: RS Vale, M King, eds. *Existential Phenomenological Alternatives for Psychology*. Oxford University Press, New York.

Cooper DR, Schindler PS (2008) *Business Research Methods*, 10th edn. McGraw-Hill, Boston.

Corbie-Smith G (1999) The continuing legacy of the Tuskegee Syphilis Study: considerations for clinical investigation. *American Journal of Medical Science* 317(1): 5–8.

Coyle ME, Smith CA, Peat B (2005) Cephalic version by moxibustion for breech presentation. *Cochrane Database Systematic Review* 2: CD003928.

Critical Appraisal Skills Programme (2006) *CASP Appraisal Tools*. Public Health Resource Unit, England. http://www.phru.nhs.uk/Doc_Links/Qualitative%20Appraisal%20Tool.pdf. Last accessed 21/09/2010.

Crombie IK (2004) *The Pocket Guide to Critical Appraisal*. BMJ Publishing Group, London.

Crotty M (1996) *Phenomenology and Nursing Research*. Churchill Livingstone, Melbourne.

Crowley P (1989) Promoting pulmonary maturity. In: I Chalmers, M Enkin, MJNC Keirse, eds. *Effective Care in Pregnancy and Childbirth*. Oxford University Press, Oxford, 746–762.

Crozier K, Macdonald S (2009) Innovation and research in midwifery. *RCM Midwives Journal*. http://www.rcm.org.uk/midwives/in-depth-papers/innovation-and-research-in-midwifery/?locale=en. Last accessed 13/04/2010.

Cutler L (2004) Ethnography. In: Bassett C, ed. *Qualitative Research in Health Care*. Whurr Publishers, London, 115–153.

Dahlen HG (2007) Reduction of perineal trauma and improved perineal comfort during and after childbirth: the perineal Warm Pack Trial. Unpublished thesis, Centre for Midwifery, Child and Family Health, Faculty of Nursing, Midwifery and Health, University of Technology, Sydney, Australia.

Dahlen HG, Ryan M, Homer C, Cooke M (2007) An Australian prospective cohort study of risk factors for severe perienal trauma during childbirth. *Midwifery* 23(2): 196–203.

Davies MB (2007) *Doing a Successful Research Project*. Palgrave Macmillan, Basingstoke.

Davies R (1996) Practitioners in their own right: an ethnographic study of the perceptions of student midwives. In: S Robinson, A Thompson, eds. *Midwives, Research and Childbirth*, vol 4. Chapman & Hall, London, 85–108.

Denscombe M (2003) *The Good Research Guide*. Open University Press, Maidenhead.

Denzin C (ed) (2000) *Handbook of Qualitative Research*, 2nd edn. Sage Publications, London.

Department of Health (2001) *Governance arrangements for NHS Research Ethics Committees*. HMSO, London. http://www.dh.gov.uk/en/Publicationsandstatistics/Publications/PublicationsPolicyAndGuidance/DH_4005727. Last accessed 9/10/2010.

Department of Health (2005) Research governance framework for health and social care, 2nd edn. Department of Health, London. http://www.dh.gov.uk/en/Publicationsandstatistics/Publications/PublicationsPolicyAndGuidance/DH_4108962. Last accessed 13/04/2010.

Dickersin K (1990) The existence of publication bias and risk factors for its occurrence. *Journal of the American Medical Association* 263(10): 1385–1389.

Dillman DA (2007) *Mail and Internet Surveys: The Tailored Design Method*, 2nd edn. Wiley, Hoboken, NJ.

Donovan P (2006) Ethnography. In: ER Cluett, R Bluff, eds. *Principles and Practice of Research in Midwifery*, 2nd edn. Elsevier, Edinburgh, 171–186.

Downe S, Gerrett D, Renfrew M (2004) A prospective randomised trial on the effect of position in the passive 2nd stage of labour on birth outcome in nulliparous women using epidural. *Midwifery* 20: 157–168.

Downe S, McCormick C, Beech BL (2001) Labour interventions associated with normal birth. *British Journal of Midwifery* 9(10): 602–606.

Downe S, Simpson L, Trafford K (2007) Expert intrapartum maternity care: a meta-synthesis. *Journal of Advanced Nursing* 57(2): 127–140.

Dykes F (2004) What are the foundations of qualitative research? In: T Lavender, G Edwards, Z Alfirevic, eds. *Demystifying Qualitative Research in Pregnancy and Child-birth*. Quay Books, Salisbury, 17–34.

Editorial commentary (2007) Reducing the play of chance using meta-analysis. *The James Lind Library*. http://www.jameslindlibrary.org.

El-Nemar A, Downe S, Small N (2005) She would help me from the heart: an ethnography of Egyptian women in labour. *Social Science & Medicine* 62: 81–92.

Emanuel E (2002) *Ethical and Regulatory Aspects of Clinical Research: Readings and Commentary*. Johns Hopkins University Press, Baltimore.

Emanuel EJ, Crouch RA, Arras JD, Moreno JD, Grady C (eds) (2003) *Ethical and Regulatory Aspects of Clinical Research*. The Johns Hopkins University Press, Baltimore.

European Association of Science Editors (EASE) (2008) EASE statement on inappropriate use of impact factors. http://www.ease.org.uk/artman2/uploads/1/EASE_statement_IFs_final.pdf. Last accessed 24/03/2010.

Evans I, Thornton H, Chalmers I (2006) *Testing Treatments: Better Research for Better Health Care*. The British Library, London.

Faragher B, Marguerie C (1998) *Essential Statistics for Medical Examinations*. Pastest, Knutsford.

Fealy GM (2008) Historical research. In: R Watson, H McKenna, S Cowman, J Keady, eds. *Nursing Research Designs and Methods*. Churchill Livingstone Elsevier, Edinburgh, 45–53.

Forsyth DR (1990) *Group dynamics*, 2nd edn. Brooks Cole, Pacific Grove, CA.

Friedman DA (1954) The graphic analysis of labor. *American Journal of Obstetrics and Gynecology* 68: 1568–1575.

Furber CM, Thomson AM (2006) Breaking the rules in baby-feeding practice in the UK: deviance and good practice? *Midwifery* 22: 365–376.

Garforth S, Garcia J (1987) Admitting – a weakness or a strength? Routine admission of a woman in labour. *Midwifery* 3(2): 10–24.

Gibbs GR (2002) *Qualitative Data Analysis Explorations with NVivo*. Open University Press, Buckingham.

Gillham B (2005) *Research Interviewing: the Range of Techniques*. Open University Press, Maidenhead.

Giorgi A (1985) Sketch of a psychological phenomenological method. In: A Giorgi, ed. *Phenomenology and Pyschological Research*. Duquesne University Press, Pittsburgh.

Glaser BG (1998) *Doing Grounded Theory: Issues and Discussions*. Sociology Press, Mill Valley, CA.

Glaser BG (2001) *The Grounded Theory Perspective: Conceptualization Contrasted with Description*. Sociology Press, Mill Valley, CA.

Glaser BG, Strauss A (1967) *Discovery of Grounded Theory. Strategies for Qualitative Research*. Sociology Press, Mill Valley, CA.

Greenhalgh T, Wengraf T (2008) Collecting stories: is it research? Is it good research? Preliminary guidance based on a Delphi Study. *Medical Education* 42: 242–247.

Griffiths F (2009) *Research Methods for Health Care Practice*. Sage Publications, London.

Grix J (2004) *The Foundations of Research*. Palgrave Macmillan, Basingstoke.

Guba EG, Lincoln YS (1994) Competing paradigms in qualitative research. In: N Denzin, YS Lincoln, eds. *Handbook of Qualitative Research*. Sage Publications, Thousand Oaks, CA, 105–111.

Guest G, Bunce A, Johnson L (2006) How many interviews are enough? *Field Methods* **18**(1): 59–82.

Haigh C (2008) Research governance and research ethics. In: R Watson, H McKenna, S Cowman, J Keady, eds. *Nursing Research*. Churchill Livingstone Elsevier, Edinburgh: 125–136.

Haigh C, Jones N (2005) An overview of the ethics of cyberspace research and the implications for nurse educators. *Nurse Education Today* **25**(1): 3–8.

Hamer S (1999) Evidence-based practice. In: S Hamer, G Collison, eds. *Achieving Evidence-Based Practice: A Handbook for Practitioners*. Balliere Tindall, London.

Hamer S, Collinson G (eds) (1999) Information sourcing. In: *Achieving Evidence-Based Practice: A Handbook for Practitioners*. Bailliere Tindall, London, Ch 4.

Hammick M (1996) Managing the ethical process. In: *Research*. Quay Books, Salisbury.

Hart C (2005) *Doing a Literature Search: A Comprehensive Guide for the Social Sciences*. Sage Publications, London.

Harvard L (2007) How to conduct an effective and valid literature search. *Nursing Times* **103**(45): 32–33.

Hasson F, Keeney S, McKenna H (2000) Research guidelines for the Delphi survey technique. *Journal of Advanced Nursing* **32**(4): 1008–1015.

Hegelund A (2005) Objectivity and subjectivity in the ethnographic method. *Qualitative Health Research* **15**: 647–668.

Hicks CM (1996) *Undertaking Midwifery Research: A Basic Guide to Design and Analysis*. Churchill Livingstone, London.

Holbrook AL, Green MC, Krosnick JA (2003) Telephone versus face-to-face interviewing of national probability samples with questionnaires. *Public Opinion Quarterly* **67**(1): 79–81.

Hollis S, Campbell F (1999) What is meant by intention to treat analysis? Survey of published randomised controlled trials. *British Medical Journal* **319**: 670–674.

Holloway I, Todres L (2006) Ethnography. In: K Gerrish, A Lacey, eds. *The Research Process in Nursing*, 5th edn. Blackwell Publishing, Oxford, 208–222.

Holloway I, Wheeler S (2002) *Qualitative Research in Nursing*, 2nd edn. Blackwell Publishing, Oxford.

Holly C (2009) Darzi's vision becomes a reality. RCM, London. http://www.rcm.org.uk/midwives/features/darzis-vision-becomes-a-reality/?locale=en. Last accessed 9/06/2010.

Home Office (2010) *British Crime Survey (July 2010)*. Home Office, UK. http://rds.homeoffice.gov.uk/rds/pdfs10/hosb1210.pdf. Last accessed 9/10/2010.

Howitt D, Cramer D (2000) Ethics in the conduct of research. In: *First Steps in Research & Statistics: a Practical Workbook for Psychology Students*. Routledge, London, Ch 3.

Hughes G (2010) A study exploring the relationship between midwives attitudes to breastfeeding and their own personal experience of breastfeeding, professional experience and professional breastfeeding education. Unpublished masters thesis, University of Chester.

Hunt S, Symonds A (1995) *The Social Meaning of Midwifery*. Macmillan, Basingstoke.

Hurwitz B, Greenhalgh T, Skultans V (2004) *Narrative Research in Health and Illness*. BMJ Publishing Group, London.

International Committee of Medical Journal Editors (1997) Uniform requirements for manuscripts submitted to biomedical journals. *Annals of Internal Medicine* **126**(1): 36–47.

Jahad AR (2000) *Randomised Controlled Trials: A User's Guide.* BMJ Publishing Group, London.

Jenner E (1798) *An Inquiry into the Causes and Effects of the Variolae or Coxpox.* Low, London.

John V, Parsons E (2006) Shadow work in midwifery: unseen and unrecognised emotional labour. *British Journal Of Midwifery* **14**(5): 266–271.

Jones K (2004) The turn to a narrative knowing of persons. In: F Rapport, ed. *New Qualitative Methodologies in Health and Social Care Research.* Routledge, New York, 35–54.

Jones S (1985) Depth interviewing. In: R Walker, ed. *Applied Qualitative Research.* Gower, Aldershot.

Kennedy H, Rousseau A, Low L (2003) An exploratory meta-synthesis of midwifery practice in the United States. *Midwifery* **19**: 203–214.

Kettle C, Hills RK, Ismail KMK (2007) Continuous versus interrupted sutures for repair of episiotomy or second degree tears. *Cochrane Database of Systematic Reviews*, Issue 4. Art No.: CD000947. DOI: 10.1002/14651858.CD000947.pub2. http://www2.cochrane.org/reviews/en/ab000947.html. Last accessed 23/03/2010.

Kettle C, Hills RK, Jones P, Darby L, Gray R, Johanson R (2002) Continuous versus interrupted perineal repair with standard or rapidly absorbed sutures after spontaneous vaginal birth: a randomised controlled trial. *Lancet* **359**(9325): 2217–2223.

Kingdon C (2005) Reflexivity: not just a qualitative methodological research tool. *British Journal of Midwifery* **13**(10): 622–627.

Kitzinger J (1994) The methodology of focus group: the importance of interaction between research participants. *Sociology of Health and Illness* **16**(12): 103–120.

Knowles-Beecher HK (1966) Ethics and clinical research. *New England Journal of Medicine* **274**: 1354–1360.

Koch T (1995) Interpretive approaches in nursing research: the influence of Husserl and Heidegger. *Journal of Advanced Nursing* **21**: 827–836.

Kopp VJ (1999) Henry Knowles-Beecher and the development of informed consent in anesthesia research. *Anesthesiology* **90**(6): 1756–1768.

Kralik D, van Loon AM (2008) Feminist research. In: R Watson, H McKenna, S Cowman, J Keady, eds. *Nursing Research Designs and Methods.* Churchill Livingstone Elsevier, Edinburgh, 35–43.

Langer E (1966) Human Experimentation: New York Verdict affirms Patients Rights. *Science* **151**(37): 663–666.

Lanoe N (2002) *Ogier's Reading Research.* Bailliere Tindall, Edinburgh, 94.

Lasagna L (1971) Decision processes in establishing the efficacy and safety of psycholtropic agents. In: J Levine, BC Sohule, L Boulhilet, eds. *Priniciples & Problems in Establishing the Efficacy of Psychotropic Agents.* US Government Printing Office, Washington DC, 29–52.

Lavender T, Kingdon C, Hart A, Gyte G, Neilson J (2005) Could a randomised trial answer the controversy relating to elective caesarean section? National survey of consultant obstetricians and heads of midwifery. *British Medical Journal* **331**: 490–491.

Leonard KL (March 2008) Is patient satisfaction sensitive to changes in the quality of care? An exploitation of the Hawthorne effect. *Journal of Health Economics* **27**(2): 444–459.

Letherby G (2003) *Feminist Research in Theory and Practice.* Open University Press, Buckingham.

Levine C (1996) Changing views of justice after Belmont: AIDS and the inclusion of 'vulnerable' subjects. In: HY Vanderpool, ed. *The Ethics of Research Involving Human Subjects: Facing the 21st Century*. University Publishing Group, Frederick, MD, 106.

Lincoln YS, Guba EG (1985) *Naturalistic Inquiry*. Sage Publications, Newbury Park, CA.

Lind J (1753) *Treatise of Scruvy*. http://www.jameslindlibrary.org/trial_records/17th_18th_Century/lind/lind_tp.html. Last accessed 12/03/2010.

Lindsay B (2007) *Understanding Research and Evidence-Based Practice*. Reflect Press, Exeter.

LoBiondo-Wood G, Haber J (Eds) (2002) *Nursing Research Methods, Critical Appraisal & Utilisation*, 5th edn. Mosby, St Louis, MO.

LoBiondo-Wood G, Haber J, Krainovich-Miller B (2002) Critical reading strategies: overview of the research process. In: G LoBiondo-Wood, J Haber, eds. *Nursing Research Methods, Critical Appraisal & Utilisation*, 5th edn. Mosby, St Louis, MO, 33–50.

Lundqvist A, Nilstun T and Dykes A (2002) Both empowered and powerless: mothers' experiences of professional care when their newborn dies. *Birth* 29(3): 192–199.

Macdonald S (ed) (2004) *Using Research in Practice A Resource for Midwives*. Royal College of Midwives, London.

Mackenzie N, Knipe S (2006) Research dilemmas: paradigms, methods and methodology. *Issues in Educational Research* 16(2): 193–205.

Macnee CL (2004) *Understanding Nursing Research*. Lippincott, Williams & Wilkins, Philadelphia, PA.

Majnemer A, Barr RG (2005) Influence of supine sleep positioning on early motor milestone acquisition. *Developmental Medicine and Child Neurology* 47(6): 370–376.

Mann T (1996) *Clinical Guidelines: Using Clinical Guidelines to Improve Patient Care within the NHS*. NHS Executive, Leeds.

Mapp T (2008) Understanding phenomenology: the lived experience. *British Journal of Midwifery* 16(5): 308–311.

Mapp T, Hudson K (2005) Feelings and fears during obstetric emergencies, Part 1. *British Journal Of Midwifery* 13(1): 30–35.

McCarthy M (2001) A century of the US Army yellow fever research. *Lancet* 357(9270): 1772.

McCormick F, Renfrew MJ (1997) *The Midwifery Research Database MIRIAD: A Sourcebook of Information about Research in Midwifery*, 3rd edn. Books for Midwives, Hale.

McHaffie HE (2000) Ethics and good practice. In: S Proctor, M Renfrew, eds. *Linking Research and Practice*. Bailliere Tindall, London.

McKee A (2003) *Textual Analysis: a Beginner's Guide*. Sage Publications, London.

McKenna H, Keeney S (2008) Delphi studies. In: R Watson, H McKenna, S Cowman, J Keady, eds. *Nursing Research Designs and Methods*. Churchill Livingstone Elsevier, Edinburgh, 251–260.

Miles MB, Huberman AM (1994) *Qualitative Data Analysis*. Routledge, London.

Mitchell M, Williams J (2007) The role of midwife–complementary therapists: data from in-depth telephone interviews. *Evidence Based Midwifery* 5(3): 93–99.

Moher D, Hopewell S, Schulz KF, Montori V, Gøtzsche PC, Devereaux PJ, Elbourne D, Egger M, Altman DG, for the CONSORT Group (2010) CONSORT 2010 Explanation and elaboration: updated guidelines for reporting parallel group randomised trial. *British Medical Journal* 340: c869.

Moher D, Schulz KF, Altman DG (2001) The CONSORT statement: revised recommendations for improving the quality of reports of parallel-group randomised trials. *Lancet* 357(9263): 1191–1194.

Moore L, Campbell R, Whelan A, Mills N, Lupton P, Misselbrook E, Frohlich J (2002) Self help smoking cessation in pregnancy: cluster randomised controlled trial. *British Medical Journal* **325**: 1383–1386.

Morgan DL (1997) *Focus Groups as Qualitative Research*. Sage Publications, London.

Morgan J (2004) Planning your research. In: T Lavender, G Edwards, Z Alfirevic, eds. *Demystifying Qualitative Research in Pregnancy and Childbirth*. Quay Books, Salisbury, 48–62.

Moustakas C (1994) *Phenomenological Research Methods*. Sage Publications, London.

Mulhall A (2003) In the field: notes on observation in qualitative research. *Journal Of Advanced Nursing* **41**(3): 306–313.

Navviba S, Abedian Z, Steen-Greaves M (2009) Effectiveness of cooling gel pads and ice packs on perineal pain. *British Journal of Midwifery* **17**(11): 724–729

NHMRC (1999) *How to Review the Evidence: Systematic Identification and Review of the Scientific Literature*. National Health & Medical Research Council, Australia.

NHMRC (2000) *How to Compare the Cost and Benefits: Evaluation of the Economic Evidence*. National Health & Medical Research Council, Australia.

NHS (2009) *NHS Evidence*. National Health Service, UK.

NICE (2002) *Principles for Best Practice in Clinical Audit*. Radcliffe Medical Press, Oxford.

NICE (2006) *Clinical Guideline CG037: Postnatal Care: Routine Postnatal Care of Women and their Babies*. http://www.nice.org.uk/CG037. Last accessed 16/09/2010.

Nixon SA, Avery MD, Savik MS (1998) Outcomes of macrosomic infants in a nurse-midwifery service. *Journal of Nurse-Midwifery* **43**(4): 280–286.

NMC (2004) *Standards of Proficiency for Pre-registration Midwifery Education*. National Midwifery Council, London.

NMC (2008) *The Code: Standards for Conduct, Performance and Ethics for Nurses and Midwives*. National Midwifery Council, London.

Noblit GW, Hare RD (1988) *Meta-Ethnography: Synthesizing Qualitative Studies*. Sage, London.

Nuremberg Code (1949) From Trials of War Criminals before the Nuremberg Military Tribunals under Control Council Law No. 10. Nuremberg, October 1946–April 1949. US GPO, 1949–1953, Washington DC.

O'Hara P (1996) *Pain Management for Health Professionals*. Chapman and Hall, London.

Olansky S, Schuman SH, Peters JJ, Smith CA, Rambo DS (1956) Untreated syphilis in the male Negro. X. Twenty years of clinical observation of untreated syphilitic and presumably nonsyphilitic groups. *Journal of Chronic Disease* **4**(2): 177–185.

Parahoo K (2000) Barriers to and facilitators of research utilization among nurses in Northern Ireland. *Journal of Advanced Nursing* **31**(1): 89–98.

Parahoo K (2006) *Nursing Research: Principles, Process and Issues*, 2nd edn. Macmillan, Basingstoke.

Parkin P (2009) *Managing Change in Healthcare Using Action Research*. Sage Publications, London.

Pincombe J, McKellar L, Grech C, Grinter E, Beresford G (2007) Registration requirements for midwives in Australia: a Delphi study. *British Journal of Midwifery* **15**(6): 372–383.

Pink S (2007) *Doing Visual Ethnography*, 2nd edn. Sage Publications, London.

Pocock SJ, Hughes MD, Lee RJ (1987) Statistical problems in the reporting of clinical trials. A survey of three medical journals. *New England Journal of Medicine* **317**: 426–432.

Polit DF, Beck CT (2006) *Essentials of Nursing Research*, 6th edn. Lippincott Williams & Wilkins, Philadelphia, PA.

Polit DF, Beck CT (2008) *Essentials of Nursing Research*, 7th edn. Lippincott Williams & Wilkins, Philadelphia, PA.

Polit DF, Beck CT, Hungler BP (2001) *Essentials of Nursing Research: Methods, Appraisal and Utilization*, 5th edn. Lippincott, Philadelphia, PA.

Price MR, Johnson M (2006) An ethnography of experienced midwives caring for women in labour. *Evidence Based Midwifery* 4(3): 101–106.

Proctor S, Renfrew M (eds) (2000) *Linking Research and Practice in Midwifery: A Guide to Evidence-Based Practice*. Bailliere Tindall, London.

RCM (2003) *Valuing Practice: A Springboard for Midwivery Education. Strategy for Education*. Royal College of Midwives, London.

RCM (2004) *Using Research in Practice: a Resource for Midwives*. Royal College of Midwives, London.

RCM (2006) *The Maze of Ethics Approval and Finding the Way! The Ethics of Research and Ethical Dilemmas whilst Undertaking Research*: Masterclass 3. Royal College of Midwives, London.

Reed W, Carroll J, Agramonte A (1901) Experimental yellow fever. *American Medicine* 2: 15–23.

Rees C (1990) The Questionnaire in Research: Clinical Research. *Nursing Standard* 4(42): 34–35.

Rees C (2003) *Introduction to Research for Midwives*, 2nd edn. Books for Midwives, Edinburgh.

Reid L (2004) Using oral history in midwifery. *British Journal of Midwifery* 12(4): 208–212.

Reil M (2007) *Understanding Action Research*. Center for Collaborative Action Research, Pepperdine University. http://cadres.pepperdine.edu/ccar/define.html. Accessed 26/08/08.

Richens Y (2002) Are midwives using research evidence in practice? *British Journal of Midwifery* 10(11): 11–16.

Riddick-Thomas NM (2009) Ethics in midwifery. In: D Frazer, M Cooper, eds. *Myles' Textbook for Midwifery*, 15th edn. Churchill-Livingstone Elsevier, Edinburgh, 57.

Roberts T (2008) Understanding grounded theory. *British Journal of Midwifery* 16(10): 679–681.

Roberts T (2009) Understanding ethnography. *British Journal of Midwifery* 17(5): 291–294.

Robinson A (2006) Phenomenology. In: ER Cluett, R Bluff, eds. *Principles and Practice of Research in Midwifery*, 2nd edn. Churchill Livingstone Elsevier, Edinburgh, 187–200.

Robinson JE (2002) Choosing your methods. In: M Tarling, L Crofts, eds. *The Essential Researcher's Handbook*. Bailliere Tindall, Edinburgh, 64–81.

Romney M (1980) Predelivery shaving: an unjustified assault. *Journal of Obstetrics and Gynaecology* 1: 33–35.

Romney M, Gordon H (1981) Is your enema really necessary? *British Medical Journal* 282: 1269–1271.

Rugg G, Petre M (2007) *A Gentle Guide to Research Methods*. Open University Press, Maidenhead.

Salmon D (1999) A feminist analysis of women's experiences of perineal trauma in the immediate post-delivery period. *Midwifery* 15(4): 247–256.

Sandelowski M, Docherty S, Emden C (1997) Qualitative meta-synthesis: issues and techniques. *Researching in Nursing and Health* **20**: 365–361.

Saunders M, Lewis P, Thornhill A (2009) *Research Methods for Business Students*, 5th edn. Pearson Education Ltd, London.

Scholl N, Mulders S, Drent R (2002) On-line qualitative market research: interviewing the world at a finger tip. *Qualitative Market Research* **5**(3): 210–223.

Schulz KF, Altman DG, Moher D, for the CONSORT Group. CONSORT 2010 Statement: updated guidelines for reporting parallel group randomised trials. *British Medical Journal* **340**: c332.

Seglen PO (1997) Why the impact factor of journals should not be used for evaluating research. *British Medical Journal* **314**(7079): 498–502.

Shields L, Winch S (2008) Ethical considerations: informed consent and protecting vulnerable populations. In: S Winch, A Henderson, L Shields, eds. *Doing Clinical Healthcare Research*. Palgrave Macmillan, Basingstoke, 23–40.

Silverman D (1997) *Interpreting qualitative data. Methods for analysing talk, text and interaction*. Sage Publications: London.

Sim J, Wright C (2000) *Research in Health Care*. Stanley Thomas Ltd, Cheltenham.

Simpson L (2007) A phenomenological exploration of midwives' accounts of midwifery expertise. Unpublished masters thesis, University of Central Lancashire, UK.

Sinclair M (2008) The Doctoral Midwifery Research Society: a concrete structure for supporting doctoral midwifery research. The Royal College of Midwives. *Evidence Based Midwifery* **6**(1): 3.

Sinclair M, Ratnaike D (2007) Writing for *Evidence Based Midwifery*. *Evidence Based Midwifery* **5**(2): 66–70.

Skulmoski GJ, Hartman FT, Krahn J (2007) The Delphi method for graduate research. *Journal of Information Technology Education* **6**: 1–21.

Sleep J, Grant A (1988) Relief of perineal pain following childbirth: a survey of midwifery practice. *Midwifery* **4**(3):118–122.

Sleep J, Grant A, Garcia J, Elbourne D, Spencer J, Chalmers I (1984) West Berkshire Perineal Management Trial. *British Medical Journal* **289**: 587–590.

Smith G (2008) Experiments. In: R Watson, H McKenna, S Cowman, J Keady, eds. *Nursing Research*. Churchill Livingstone Elsevier, Edinburgh, 189–198.

Sorrell JM, Redmond GM (1995) Interviews in qualitative nursing research: differing approaches for ethnographic and phenomenological studies. *Journal of Advanced Nursing* **21**: 1117–1122.

Stapleton H, Kirkham M, Thomas G (2002) Qualitative study of evidence-based leaflets in maternity care. *British Medical Journal* **324**: 639.

Steen M (2004) Women's experiences of pain and healing following perineal trauma after childbirth. Unpublished thesis, Leeds Metropolitan University, England.

Steen M (2007) Well-being & beyond. *RCM Midwives Journal* **10**(3): 116–119.

Steen MP (2002) A randomised controlled trial to evaluate the effectiveness of localised cooling treatments in alleviating perineal trauma: The APT Study. *MIDIRS Midwifery Digest* **12**(3): 373–376.

Steen MP (2005) 'I can't sit down' – easing genital tract trauma. *British Journal of Midwifery* **13**(5): 311–314.

Steen MP (2010) Structured interview schedules: diet & nutrition. Research dissertation, MW6005, University of Chester, UK.

Steen M, Anker J (2008) Postures and Positions in Labour: Best Practice. Conference presentation. National Primary Care Conference, NEC Birmingham. http://chester-rep.openrepository.com/cdr/handle/10034/48456. Last accessed 24/03/2010.

Steen M, Calvert J (2007) A follow up study of women's experiences of using self administration homeopathic remedies. *British Journal of Midwifery* 15: 7.

Steen MP, Cooper KJ (1997) A tool for assessing perineal trauma. *Journal of Wound Care* 6(9): 432–436.

Steen MP, Cooper KJ (1998) Cold therapy and perineal wounds: too cool or not too cool? *British Journal of Midwifery* 6(9): 572–579.

Steen MP, Cooper KJ (1999) A new device for the treatment of perineal wounds. *Journal of Wound Care* 8(2): 87–90.

Steen M, Kingdon C (2008a) Vaginal or Caesarean delivery? How research has turned breech birth around. *Evidence Based Midwifery* 6(3): 95–99.

Steen M, Kingdon C (2008b) Breech birth: reviewing the evidence for external cephalic version. *Evidence-Based Midwifery* 6(4): 126–129.

Steen M, Macdonald S (2008) A review of baby skin care. Midwives online, Aug/Sept, Royal College of Midwives. http://www.rcm.org.uk/midwives/in-depth-papers/a-review-of-baby-skin-care/

Steen M, Marchant P (2007) Ice packs and cooling gel pads versus no localised treatment for relief of perineal pain: a randomised controlled trial. *Evidence Based Midwifery* 5(1): 16–22.

Steen MP, Marchant PR (2001) Alleviating Perineal Trauma: the APT Study. *RCM Midwives Journal* 4(8): 256–259.

Steen M, Briggs M, King D (2006) Alleviating postnatal perineal trauma. To cool or not to cool? *British Journal of Midwifery* 14(5): 304–308.

Steen MP, Cooper KJ, Marchant P, Griffiths-Jones M, Walker J (2000) A randomised controlled trial to compare the effectiveness of ice packs and Epifoam with cooling maternity gel pads at alleviating postnatal perineal trauma. *Midwifery* 16(1): 48–55.

Steen M, Rigby K, Downe S, Fisher D, Burgess A, Davies J (2008) Involving father in maternity care: Best Practice. NMC Annual Conference, Manchester. http://chester-rep.openrepository.com/cdr/handle/10034/48457. Last accessed 24/03/2010.

Steen-Greaves M, Downe S, Graham-Kevan N (2009) Men and women's perceptions and experiences of attending an abusive behaviour management programme. *Evidence Based Midwifery* 7(4): 128–135.

Strauss A, Corbin J (1997) *Grounded Theory in Practice*. Sage Publications, Thousand Oaks, CA.

Strauss A, Corbin J (1998) *Basics Of Qualitative Research Techniques and Procedures for Developing Grounded Theory*, 2nd edn. Sage Publications, Thousand Oaks, CA.

Swetnam D (2004) *Writing your Dissertation: The Bestselling Guide to Planning, Preparing, and Presenting, First Class Work*. 3rd edn. Cromwell Press Ltd, Trowbridge.

Thomas BG (2006) 'Making a difference': midwives' experiences of caring for women. *Evidence Based Midwifery* 4(3): 83–88.

Thompson FE (2003) The practice setting: site of ethical conflict for some mothers and midwives. *Nursing Ethics* 10(6): 588–601.

Todres L, Holloway I (2004) Descriptive phenomenology: life world as evidence. In: F Rapport, ed. *New Qualitative Methodologies in Health & Social Care Research*. Routledge, London, 79–98.

Tohotoa J, Maycock B, Hauck YL, Howat P, Burns S, Binns CW (2009) Dads make a difference: an exploratory study of paternal support for breastfeeding in Perth, Western Australia. *International Breastfeeding Journal* 4: 15.

Tuckman BW, Jenson MAC (1977) Development sequences in small groups. *Psychological Bulletin* 63: 384–399.

United States Holocaust Memorial Museum (2008) Trials of War Criminals before the Nuremburg Military Tribunals under Control Council Law No 10. Nuremburg October 1946–April 1949. http://www.ushmm.org/research/doctors/codeptx/htm. Last accessed 23/09/2009.

University of Chester (2010) *Guide to Postgraduate Research Degrees (MPhil & PhD).* University of Chester, Chester.

Van Kaam A (1966) *Existential Foundations of Psychology.* Duquesne University Press, Pittsburgh.

Van Teijlingen, E, Ireland J (2003) Research interviews in midwifery. *Midwives* 6(6): 260–263.

Varcoe C, Rodney P, McCormick J (2003) Health care relationships in context: an analysis of three ethnographies. *Qualitative Health Research* 13: 957–973.

Walliman N (2005) *Your Undergraduate Dissertation: The Essential Guide to Success.* Sage Publications, London.

Walsh D (1996) Evidence-based practice: whose evidence and on what basis? *British Journal of Midwifery* 4(9): 454–457.

Walsh D, Downe S (2005) Meta-synthesis method for qualitative research: a literature review. *Journal of Advanced Nursing* 50: 204–211.

Walsh D, Downe S (2006) Catching the wind: appraising the quality of qualitative research. *Midwifery* 22: 108–119.

Walsh M, Wiggens L (2003) *Introduction to Research Foundations in Nursing and Health Care.* Nelson Thornes Ltd, London.

Walters AJ (1995) The phenomenological movement: implications for nursing research. *Journal of Advanced Nursing* 22: 791–799.

Walton C, Yiannousiz K, Gatsby H (2005) Promoting midwifery-led care within an obstetric-led unit. *British Journal of Midwifery* 13(12): 750–755.

Warmel M (1996) Materials and methods for perineal repair following childbirth. *British Journal of Midwifery* 4(2): 65.

Waterman H, Hope K (2008) Action research. In: R Watson, H McKenna, S Cowman, J Keady, eds. *Nursing Research.* Churchill Livingstone Elsevier, Edinburgh, 211–220.

Watson R, Keady J (2008) The nature and language of nursing research. In: R Watson, H McKenna, S Cowman, J Keady, eds. *Nursing Research.* Churchill Livingstone Elsevier, Edinburgh, 3–12.

Webb C (2003) An introduction to guidelines on reporting qualitative research. *Journal of Advanced Nursing* 42(6): 544–545.

Wilkins C (2006) A qualitative study exploring the support needs of first-time mothers on their journey towards intuitive parenting. *Midwifery* 22(2): 169–180.

Williams A (2008) Ethnography. In: R Watson, H McKenna, S Cowman, J Keady, eds. *Nursing Research.* Churchill Livingstone Elsevier, Edinburgh, 243–250.

Williams J (2006) Why women choose midwifery: a narrative analysis of motivations and understandings in a group of first-year student midwives. *Evidence Based Midwifery* 4(2): 46–52.

World Health Organization (2003) *Managing Newborn Problems: A Guide for Doctors, Nurses and Midwives.* Department of Reproductive Health and Research. World Health Organization, Geneva. http://www.who.int/reproductivehealth/publications/maternal_perinatal_health/9241546220/en/index.html. Last accessed 16/09/2010.

World Medical Association (2008) WMA Declaration of Helsinki Ethical Principles for Medical Research involving Human Subjects. http://www.wma.net/en/30publications/10policies/b3/index.html. Last accessed 17/04/2010.

Wynne-Jones JA (2008) The development and implementation of a framework for best practice with regard to nursing/midwifery shift handover. Masters Thesis, Auckland University of Technology, New Zealand. http://aut.researchgateway.ac.nz/bitstream/10292/656/6/WynneJonesJ.pdf. Last accessed 29/03/2010.

Yinger R (1985) Journal writing as a learning tool. *Volta Review* **87**(5): 21–33.

Index

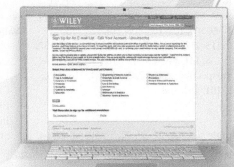

Printed and bound by CPI Group (UK) Ltd, Croydon, CR0 4YY

09/10/2024

14571430-0003